# Finding Life's Secret Sauce

# Finding Life's Secret Sauce

*How to Fit Good Food, Fitness, and Fun
into your Crazy, Busy Schedule*

## MELINDA HINSON NEELY

New York

# Finding Life's Secret Sauce

How to fit good food, fitness, and fun into your crazy busy schedule

Cover Design by:  Rachel Lopez - Racehl@r2cdesign

Photographs by Barb Bergeson - www.barbbergeson.com

ISBN 978-1-60037-710-5

Library of Congress Control Number: 2009936513

# MORGAN · JAMES
### THE ENTREPRENEURIAL PUBLISHER

Morgan James Publishing
1225 Franklin Ave., STE 325
Garden City, NY 11530-1693
Toll Free 800-485-4943
www.MorganJamesPublishing.com

In an effort to support local communities, raise awareness and funds, Morgan James Publishing donates one percent of all book sales for the life of each book to Habitat for Humanity. Get involved today, visit **www.HelpHabitatForHumanity.org**.

# *Dedication*

To the four Bubs, my life's secret sauce.

And Shelby, whose secret sauce was life itself.

# Table of Contents

# *Preface*

**Reasons not to read this book:**

I'm not a doctor.

I am not a health professional of any sort, for that matter.

I'm not a movie star (whom we all know are experts on pretty much *every* topic, of course).

I'm no Donald Trump or self-made millionaire (not yet, anyway).

I am not an expert on well-being, and certainly not qualified to tell a *bona fide* grown-up like you how to live your life.

**Reasons it might be worth reading:**

Actually, these are the same reasons why you might just get something out of this book.

**I am neither a doctor nor a health professional.** That means I can explain things in a language ordinary people use and understand. I won't throw out a bunch of medical terminology that needs to be decoded or researched. I won't even give you a pill to make it all better—you'll need to work a little harder for my prescriptions to work.

**I'm not a movie star.** I don't have an entourage of trainers, health professionals and beauticians following me around, helping me feel and look better. Whatever I have managed to accomplish in the way of healthier living has been the result of my own discipline, desire, willingness to experiment and more than one misstep along the way.

**I'm no Donald Trump.** What I've learned and am about to share with you has not made me wealthy or famous. I've always worked hard to make a good living, and unfortunately, did not inherit a trust fund or luck out on a lottery ticket. So when I've incorporated healthy habits into the routine, I've had to do so the good old fashioned way—while juggling meetings, relocations, business trips, some failed relationships and (finally!) a successful marriage and children.

**I am not an expert on well-being or a guru with all the answers**. On the contrary, I am a regular person just like you with good intentions and weaknesses and insights, who knows what it's like to achieve a great big goal as well as what it's like to get blown off course when life happens.

I have been through the ups and downs of gaining/losing weight and have safely and healthfully maintained my current weight for years, without any special diets or expensive programs. And I run marathons, run a business, enjoy my family and friends, and have somehow managed to make it all work pretty darn well. Staying healthy is not a diet pill, surgical procedure or trip to the spa; it's a life-long commitment to better habits.

Ask my friends. They'll tell you, as they tell me, that I have inspired them over the years to live healthier lives. It's thanks to their encouragement that I found myself writing this book and sharing my cure for the wellness blues. Whether you can swallow it whole or digest it in small doses, I hope you find a secret sauce that lasts a lifetime.

EAT UP

I love to eat. And I love to eat *good* food. And I decided a long time ago I had better figure out a lifestyle which did not necessitate starvation. I want mealtimes to be a special and enjoyable part of my day, and a guilt-free experience I can share with friends and family. Not a fat-free, lettuce-filled onslaught of deprivation.

SHAPE UP

I don't always love exercising when I'm in the middle of it, but I love how workouts make me feel after they're over. Without workouts, I would have trouble sleeping, I would have a far less optimistic outlook on life and I'd wear a much larger pants size.

## LIVE IT UP

In my forties, I've come to appreciate how so many aspects of my life influence my health and well-being. Family, friends, profession and entertainment—each of these plays an important part in making me a happier, more whole person.

## SUMMED UP

I have by no means perfected the formula of good health and happiness. It's a work in progress and I'm still learning from my mistakes.

But I've also discovered some real-life tricks for eating well, staying fit and keeping life adventurous. And if I can do that, no doubt you can, too.

# Eat Up!

Ain't nothin' in the world that I like better
Than bacon & lettuce & homegrown tomatoes
Up in the mornin' out in the garden

Get you a ripe one don't get a hard one
Plant 'em in the spring eat 'em in the summer
All winter with out 'em's a culinary bummer
I forget all about the sweatin' & diggin'
Everytime I go out & pick me a big one

Homegrown tomatoes homegrown tomatoes
What'd life be without homegrown tomatoes
Only two things that money can't buy
That's true love & homegrown tomatoes

You can go out to eat & that's for sure
But it's nothin' a homegrown tomato won't cure
Put 'em in a salad, put 'em in a stew
You can make your very own tomato juice
Eat 'em with eggs, eat 'em with gravy
Eat 'em with beans, pinto or navy
Put 'em on the site put 'em in the middle
Put a homegrown tomato on a hotcake griddle

Guy Clark, "Homegrown Tomatoes"

# THE SKINNY ON SKINNY

We are brainwashed to believe that being skinny is the pinnacle of health and well-being. From books to magazines to movies to fashion runways, being skinny and looking good are what it's all about. Why is the message always about slimming down, losing weight and having perfect abs?

I actually just received an email announcement about a "Celebrity Slim Down" from a reputable health publisher. Sure, we see photos of famous stars (like Gwyneth Paltrow or Demi Moore or Kate Hudson) looking like a million dollars three weeks after having a baby and say, "Why can't I do that?"

But movie stars have resources—and pressures—we don't. A million dollar figure is not a realistic goal for those of us who juggle work, family, fitness and fun—without a slew of chefs, assistants or personal trainers to get us through our day.

More importantly, there is more to life than thin thighs. You can be just as happy and healthy wearing a size 8 as a size 2. Inner beauty and health are the gifts that last a lifetime. It's not all about being skinny, contrary to popular opinion.

I grew up as the lone tomboy in a house full of girls. Some of my most exciting memories as a child were walking across the top of the monkey bars at age seven and beating Williams Poindexter in a 50-yard dash in our back yard a few years after that.

In junior high, I grew to my current height yet failed develop in other ways most 13-year old girls do. I started running, though I wasn't very good, and ate fruits and vegetables because I really liked them. Even when I started filling out in high school, I remained pretty lean, in part due to playing basketball.

Despite being in good shape, my friends and I spent countless hours comparing who had the thinnest legs, flattest stomach or most appealing butt. And despite having perfectly normal body weights, we still felt compelled to go on crazy liquid and all-fruit diets. It's hard to believe, but society is even more obsessed with skinniness today than it was back then.

When I went to college, I gained more than my fair share of "freshman weight." Besides experimenting with how many beers I could consume in a single outing, I ate a lot, too. I'd order a Domino's pizza and eat the entire thing. Or bake a package of muffins and down them all. After joining a sorority, it only got worse. The cooks at our sorority house whipped up some of the finest, and most fattening, southern dishes imaginable. And guess who snuck around late at night for leftover desserts when she was still awake studying?

Coupled with my new overeating habit was a complete halt in exercise. I didn't play any varsity or club sports in college, so my fitness declined as my shirt size increased. Even when I did start to jog again, I found it difficult to shake the weight I'd gained. And the more I obsessed about my ever-growing figure, the more I couldn't stop eating. It was a vicious cycle. By the time I graduated, my weight had jumped 25 pounds from day one at school.

It took me a long time to drop those 25 pounds, almost five years, in fact. Fad diets were not the solution. Trying to skip a meal here or cut some calories there didn't do the trick either. Even my religiously regular daily runs didn't result in the figure I wanted. And at the time I didn't even have a spouse or kids to blame for my condition. I was a single, working professional with all the time in the world to take care of myself. Right?

It wasn't until I wholeheartedly and permanently embraced better health habits that I gradually lost the weight. It meant kicking the southern diet and opting for a healthier one. It took moderation in eating (and beer drinking). Though I continued to run, I integrated new activities into the mix. I pursued a graduate degree and career, while finding the time to eat right and stay fit—and keep my life in balance (usually, at least).

My figure is by no means perfect, nor is my lifestyle any less hectic than it ever was. In fact, I am now running a business and raising a child at the same time I am dealing with the issues gravity and aging have thrust upon me (a joyful experience, I might add).

Still, since the age of 27, I have kept the weight off, with minor fluctuations here and there, most notably when my belly expanded during pregnancy. Not only do I feel better about myself, I just *feel better*. *This*, to me, is the pinnacle of health and wellness.

I firmly believe that permanent changes in well-being—including weight control—are attainable without turning your life upside down. Regardless of how much you work or what you do for a living. Whether you are married or single. If or when you ever have kids.

And what may sound counterintuitive to a focus on losing weight and being skinny, well-being starts with good food.

# EXPERIENCE THE ART OF COOKING

I am amazed at how many people prefer to avoid the kitchen. My dear friend Dawn claims her best meal is the Chinese take-out she picks up on her way home from the office. After all, who can tell the difference when it's sitting on fine China?

The catch-22 is a lack of control over what you consume. That's why my first recommendation to anyone wanting to eat better, more healthy food is simple:

**Learn how to cook.**

Cooking is not that difficult, especially if you ever braved the chemistry labs of college like I did. You don't have to be a gourmet chef to cook good food. Rachel Ray has proven you don't have to spend hours in the kitchen to have a delicious, nutritious dinner. Even the best of chefs insist that the secret is using fresh ingredients, not talent. And if you don't know how to fix it yourself, there's now TV cooking shows to suit anyone's cooking style. If you don't have any cookbooks, there are enough recipes online to fill a million libraries. Not to mention videos that show you how to do pretty much anything (except boil water, a talent you can likely master on your own).

My parents divorced when I was a small child, and I wanted to alleviate my mom's heavy load of responsibilities by helping out in the kitchen. As such, I made delicacies such as meatloaf and spaghetti when I was only eight years old. I treasured my first *Betty Crocker for Kids* cookbook.

As I broached the teenage years, my repertoire expanded to include fine treats like brownies and home-made cinnamon rolls. Though these recipes did not exactly pave the way to a flat tummy and toned thighs, at least they taught me how to measure ingredients and turn on an oven. And more importantly, they introduced me to the joys of sharing food with people you love. Even in those years, my friends and I socialized around kitchen activities.

I continued to cook throughout my twenties; but unfortunately, the meals weren't always the healthiest. I had been brought up a southern girl, after all, and as such I used too much mayonnaise and butter in all the main dishes I prepared, and loads of sugar in my desserts.

As much as I hate to admit it, it took two unsuccessful relationships to open my eyes to the benefits of a better diet. What were the chances I'd get involved with two men in a row with ridiculously high cholesterol, both of whom liked to cook and were great at cutting the fat and calories? Despite the fact those relationships didn't have staying power for me, the healthier cooking and eating habits did. And that was far better than facing a health condition of my own, which is often the motivation behind many people's change in habits.

Don't wait until something's wrong to start eating better and cooking healthier. Start now and *prevent* problems. Here are a few tips to jumpstart a new you in the kitchen.

### Start with something easy.
If you are using a recipe, read it from start to finish. If you tally up the minutes it takes to do this and that, and the total is over an hour, scratch that recipe and try something else. After all, after a long day of work, who wants to spend hours slaving over a stove anyway? Most online recipes give you guidance on how easy or difficult a dish is to make—a great time-saver for chefs of all levels.

### Read the recipe from start to finish.
This can't be said enough times. I can't tell you how many dishes I have ruined because I was in too big of a hurry to read all the way through the recipe. I would dive in and start doing one thing only to realize I should have done something else first. Thinking through what you need to do before you start doing it can save time and prevent disasters.

### It may not be as easy as it looks on TV.
Celebrity chefs have lots of helpers behind the scenes and an extra batch of everything in the stove at all times.

**Learn how to use a knife.**

Chopping usually takes more time than anything else in cooking, so "ease of doing" in a recipe description can be deceiving if you don't know how to use a knife. Take a class, ask a professional for lessons, or at least watch a video or two to learn a few chopping and slicing techniques. Hopefully you will avoid the same scars I have on my fingers.

**If you don't know how to do something, ask.**

Some culinary skills can be rather difficult to learn—such as filleting a big piece of tenderloin, butterflying a chicken, or poaching a whole fish. Maybe your hang-up is as simple as roasting a vegetable or cutting a clove of garlic, but don't be afraid to ask for help. Everyone who has mastered these skills didn't know how to do it at some point in their lives.

**Use fresh ingredients.**

Regardless of what you are fixing, it'll taste better if it's fresh. Better yet, grow your own vegetables and herbs. Not only do they taste better, but they might save you a dollar or two. (And gardening is very therapeutic as well.)

**Read cookbooks.**

Really read them, and not just the recipes. Many of my cookbooks have been incredibly helpful at explaining how to prepare a dish, substitute ingredients or grow spices in your garden. The first time I made gnocchi, it was a total flop. Then I read in one of Jamie Oliver's cookbooks that making gnocchi is tricky and difficult. He followed that assertion with suggestions to prevent problems. That's the kind of cookbook I like!

**Be inventive.**

I used to have a total panic attack (especially when I was cooking for others) if I forgot to buy an essential ingredient. I'd race out to the nearest store and spend way too much money for a half-teaspoon of some rare spice I wouldn't use again for months. Now admittedly, if you are baking a dessert and don't have butter and sugar, you might have a problem on your hands. But if the recipe calls for fava beans and you can't find them anywhere in town, search online for a reasonable substitute. You won't offend the recipe's author and you may even end up with a dish that's better than the original.

## Cut and see.

How many times have you overcooked an expensive piece of beef or fish? Though some fish are more forgiving than others, nothing makes me madder than spending $30/pound for a fresh piece of King Salmon and then cooking it too long. Once it's overcooked, it's too late. So avoid the problem altogether and check earlier. Cut a slice right there in the middle of whatever it is you are cooking and see if it's done. Wouldn't you rather see a knife mark and eat a delicious meal than gnaw on a perfect-looking piece of something that is ruined?

## Have fun.

Like anything in life, if it's all work and no fun, cooking will not be contributing to your overall well-being. So have a glass of wine while you go at it. Or maybe invite a friend over to help. Or (my personal favorite) ask your spouse to do the part you don't like doing (like grating cheese or chopping veggies). There are a number of ways to spice up the cooking experience. And the cooking experience you gain will broaden your repertoire for entertaining, eating well and feeling good.

# *UNDERSTAND YOUR HERITAGE*

Whether it's your eating habits, table manners or view of the world, you never really shake your heritage. I haven't lived in the South for 15 years, but this region of the country will always be an important part of who I am. After all, anyone who attended a "white gloves and party manners class" at the age of seven isn't likely to forget her heritage.

Like other parts of southern culture, many of its dishes are delightfully indulgent. From sweet tea to fried oysters to hush puppies, I am convinced that southern delicacies cannot be replicated in other parts of the country. Where else but the South would you find amazing home-made meals in a college sorority house? No wonder I gained that freshman 25!

I realized in my mid-twenties and into my thirties that the southern diet was not only influencing my weight, but my overall well-being, too. Fresh fish is one of my favorite foods in the world, but I'd never eaten it any way except fried until I ventured further north to live. Dishes prepared in the south are often high in fat, particularly those served in restaurants. That is one reason why they taste so good. But buyer beware! Fat and calories have costly consequences.

I can't completely give up my hometown cuisine, especially when I travel back to visit. In addition to the other tips I'll share later, I've learned to tweak some of my favorite regional dishes so I can cook them at home with a clear conscience. The tweaks are pretty simple:

- Use less mayonnaise.
- If the recipe says to sauté something in ¼" of oil, use a few tablespoons instead.
- Use less bacon. Many recipes call for bacon and lots of it. I admit bacon tastes great, but it doesn't take a whole lot to flavor foods. A little does the trick just as well.

# Recipes

We all grew up accustomed to some sort of regional style, some healthier than others. By learning how to cook and thinking about the ingredients, we can almost always find a way to transform our most-loved down-home gut-busters into healthier alternatives that still satisfy. Here's one example of how I have managed over the years to cut back on fat and calories from a traditional recipe. My modifications are in italics and parentheses.

## Shrimp and Grits

This recipe came from the late Bill Neal, former owner and chef of Crook's Corner in Chapel Hill—my favorite restaurant when I attended the University of North Carolina. I'll start with the original ingredients and make suggestions on where to cut back to make it healthier. This dish serves four.

> 1 batch cheese grits (see recipe below)
> 1 pound fresh shrimp
> 6 slices bacon (*2–3 slices are plenty*)
> Peanut oil
> 2 cups sliced white button mushrooms
> 1 cup minced scallions
> 1 large glove garlic, peeled and minced
> 4 teaspoons lemon juice
> Tabasco sauce
> Salt and pepper
> 2 tablespoons fresh parsley

1. Prepare the grits (see below) and hold in a warm place.
2. Peel the shrimp, rinse and pat dry.
3. Dice the bacon and sauté in a skillet until the edges of the bacon are brown, but the bacon is not crisp. Remove from heat and drain on paper towels; then crumble.
4. Add enough peanut oil to make a layer of fat ⅛" thick to the same skillet. (*Drain out almost all of the bacon grease, leaving bits for flavor, and then add just enough peanut or olive oil to coat the bottom of the pan.*)

5. When the oil is hot, add the shrimp in an even layer. Turn the shrimp as soon as they start to turn pink; add the mushrooms and sauté, stirring, about four minutes.
6. Add the scallions and garlic. Heat and stir about one minute more. Then season with lemon juice, a dash or two of Tabasco sauce, salt and pepper to taste and parsley.
7. Divide the grits evenly between four plates. Spoon the shrimp over, sprinkle with bacon (*or leave off the bacon to make a bit healthier*), and serve immediately.

## Cheese Grits

> 1 cup quick (not instant) grits
> 2 cups water
> 2 cups milk (*1% or skim milk*)
> 1 cup cheddar cheese
> ¼ cup grated parmesan cheese
> 4 tablespoons butter (*make it 1 tablespoon*)
> ½ teaspoon salt
> ⅛ teaspoon white pepper

1. Cook the grits according to the package directions.
2. Turn off heat and add remaining ingredients. Stir until just mixed.
3. If you don't serve the grits immediately, then cover and remove from heat. If the grits get too thick while sitting, just add a little milk and reheat.

## Hoppin' John

This is a must-eat on New Years' Day to bring good fortune to your family in the coming year. As southern as this dish may be, my native-of-Michigan spouse loves it, any day of the year. Here are the ingredients you'll need to get started:

> Dried black-eyed peas
> Bacon
> Rice
> Cheddar cheese
> Green onions
> Tomatoes
> Tabasco sauce

Even though some recipes for Hoppin' John allow for canned black-eyed peas, I highly recommend starting from dried ones. Start by soaking them according to the directions on the package. After soaking and draining the peas, fry up a one to three slices of bacon in a large pan (the same one in which you'll cook the peas). Leave the bacon grease in the pan and then add the bacon back in when cooking the peas. Other than this bacon step, follow the directions just as the package says.

To complete Hoppin' John, prepare three or more cups of cooked rice (white or brown tastes great). For the garnish, prepare about a cup of sliced green onions (green parts included), another cup of chopped tomatoes, and one to two cups of grated cheddar cheese.

For each serving, start with a scoop or two of rice, another scoop or two of peas, and then pile the onions, tomato and cheese according to taste. I personally go for lots of everything! Depending on your threshold for heat, you might wish to add a dash or two of Tabasco sauce.

My family loves Hoppin' John with cornbread on the side. Though the southern cornbread recipes are, of course, the best, they are typically laden with Crisco or lard. If this is an ingredient you'd like to avoid in your diet as much as I do, then just use the recipe on the side of a standard corn meal package.

## Chicken Divan

> 2–3 heads broccoli, chopped (about 3 cups, enough to cover the bottom of a 9" × 13" baking dish)
>
> 2 chicken breasts (it's okay to substitute leftover chicken or turkey)
>
> Lemon

Simmer chicken breasts about 20–30 minutes until nearly cooked. Alternatively, you could pan-fry them—do whatever is easiest and most convenient. Season the raw broccoli with a little fresh lemon, then place chicken over broccoli.

> Combine:
>
> 1 can cream of mushroom soup (*I use the low-fat or no-fat variety*)
>
> ½ cup mayonnaise (*¼ cup is enough*)
>
> 1 tablespoon sour cream (*low-fat sour cream works great*)
>
> 1 tablespoon fresh lemon juice
>
> ⅛ teaspoon curry powder

Pour mixture over broccoli and chicken then grate about one cup of cheddar cheese on top (*reduced-fat cheese tastes great*). If you have some saltines in your pantry, crush about ½ cup and pour on top of the cheese. If you don't have them, the dish will still be fine.

Bake at 350 degrees for about 30 minutes and serve.

# ADOPT A FEW EASY HABITS

A friend once told me, "Take a long, hard look at your future spouse's parents. Your spouse will become those people one day." And though I have come to appreciate the merit of her words—we do tend to become our parents—I also think there's an even better saying which fairly represents a person:

**You are what you eat.**

There's no getting around it. If you don't eat well, you don't feel well. That's right! If you eat junk food, you are going to feel like crap.

Years ago when my family came to my house for Christmas, I prepared a huge feast. Alongside the turkey and dressing sat a platter of steamed broccoli. One family member who had grown up eating the fine cuisine of Memphis, Tennessee, reacted as if I had committed some kind of crime. "What is this?" he asked, with a grimace I'd never seen.

If you have grown up seeing and eating mushy broccoli disguised in a cloak of butter and cheese, you've adapted your tastes accordingly. But just as easily as you grew accustomed to one way of eating, you can easily change to another. And believe it or not, as your body adjusts to healthier food, you will lose your desire to go back to the old ways.

Try these simple hints to jumpstart new habits.

## Use less butter.

When you serve bread with meals, try eating it without butter. Just try. And if you absolutely can't do it, then substitute olive oil. Better yet, don't eat bread at all. It adds a lot of calories without adding many, if any, nutrients.

Also, if you are cooking most any dish at home—from fish to veggies to casseroles—try using less butter than you have in the past. If you are pan-frying fish and a recipe suggests an entire stick of butter, use half a stick. My rule of thumb is that any main dish with more than four tablespoons of butter is overdoing it—unless you are feeding an army. Usually you can't tell the difference, and even if anyone does notice, it will still taste great with the reduced amount.

Even in baking you can experiment with less oil and butter. Sometimes it works and sometimes it doesn't. But if a recipe has an extraordinarily humongous amount of fat, it might well taste just as good with less of it.

## Use olive oil instead of butter.

As Rachel Ray likes to say at least twenty times in every 30-minute show: "EVOO." That's right—extra virgin olive oil. My recommendation is to use high-quality olive oil that is first cold pressed. Skip the extra light version that has no flavor at all. First cold pressed is processed less, closer to its natural state, and therefore more flavorful. I tend to use the more expensive brands when eating it fresh (for dipping bread or making salad dressing) and the less expensive brands when preparing cooked dishes.

The health benefits of olive oil are rarely disputed. Olive oil is composed of monounsaturated fatty acids which control LDL ("bad") cholesterol levels while raising HDL ("good") levels. Studies have even shown that olive oil protects against heart disease.

But the best part is that olive oil tastes really good. Chef Jamie Oliver makes most of his mashed potatoes with olive oil and salt only. You should try them some time. You'll be amazed at how good they taste. And they are so much better for you than ones loaded with butter and sour cream.

## Don't cook your vegetables to death.

My grandmother used to have a garden filled with wonderful green beans and peas and other vegetables. Then she would turn them to mush by cooking them for hours, accompanied with bacon grease, lard or a ham hock. She actually kept a big can of bacon grease sitting by the stove to use for a variety of dishes! I don't fault my grandmother; that was the way it was done in her time and region of the country. But we know better now, so it's time to adjust our habits.

Buy fresh vegetables whenever possible—the fresher and more natural the better. Canned vegetables and even frozen ones have valuable nutrients removed. When cooking them at home, try to steam or boil then as briefly as possible. The more you cook them, the more nutrients are lost. Add a small amount of butter if you must, but experiment with olive oil, spices and lemon. They'll taste great, and you'll appreciate the flavor of the vegetable versus the flavor of fat.

Raw diets are popular these days for a reason. Though healthy, I find this style of eating a bit extreme, and I don't want to inconvenience myself and others just to satisfy stringent diet requirements. So I tend to cook my veggies briefly, preserving nutrients, with no sacrifice in taste.

## Go red, not white.

Though I talk about this subject at greater length in the eating out chapter, the same theory holds true at home. Dishes made with red sauces are usually healthier than ones made with white sauces. Guess how white sauces are made? With cream and butter. It's hard to get around it. I have tried to substitute milk in the place of cream; sometimes it works and sometimes you are left with a soupy, lumpy mess that no one wants to touch. Again, a little experimentation is worth the effort.

## Don't deep fry.

This is an easy rule. Just stop eating deep fried food, whether you are at home or at a restaurant. The rule is much easier to follow at home, admittedly. Doesn't it seem wasteful to use an entire bottle of oil for one dish anyway?

## Watch the cheese.

This is a tough one for me because I love cheese in almost any shape, size or form. Cheese contains calcium and other essential nutrients such as calcium, phosphorus, zinc, vitamin A, riboflavin, vitamin B12 and high-quality protein. However, cheese can also be high in saturated fat, calories and cholesterol. When consumed in high quantities, cheese can add on the pounds if you're not careful. Moderation is what it's all about, and cheese is no exception to the rule. A few hints:

- Softer cheeses such as feta, fresh goat cheese and Neufchatel have about a third less fat than hard cheeses like cheddar.
- Flavorful cheeses like Parmesan, Gorgonzola and extra sharp cheddar can be used in smaller quantities, because a little goes a long way.
- Part-skim ricotta and low-fat cottage cheese have enough fat to still taste good. Reduced-fat cheddar isn't bad, either, but I prefer substituting a smaller dose of a stronger cheese, especially if you are baking with it.

**Use low-fat substitutes whenever possible.**
Especially if you are making casseroles, it's hard to tell whether you used low-fat sour cream instead of the full-fat version, even more so if you buy a good brand (I find the private label brands to be a bit runny). Though I have removed cream of mushroom or cream of chicken soups from most of the dishes I prepare, on the rare occasions when I do use them (like chicken divan), I use the fat-free versions.

Mayonnaise is the exception—I don't really like reduced-fat mayonnaise and would prefer to use less of the real thing than switch to a poorer tasting version.

**Don't buy junk.**
When I was single and had finally lost the freshman 25, I completely weaned myself off potato chips and candy. And this was not because I possessed an amazing sense of willpower. I simply didn't buy junk food I knew I didn't need to eat, except for minor relapses during especially frenzied weeks of PMS. Why have boxes of brownie and cake mix in the

cupboard when they cry in need of preparation (which I am convinced they do in a subliminal voice)? If it's out of sight, it's out of mind.

Having a husband and child has made it considerably more challenging to keep junk food at bay, as they both want a week supply of Tostitos, Cheese Nips and Oreos in the panty at all times. But as long as no one buys Kettle Chips, I can generally control myself. (And you can keep working on healthier snack alternatives for everyone else, too).

# STOP COUNTING CALORIES

I must preface this chapter by suggesting that I do not own an iPhone (not yet, anyway). But from what I have seen, iPhones come with enough applications to help even the most calorie-phobic soul keep track of their intake. But do they really help?

I spent a lot of time in high school, college and my early twenties obsessing over the caloric content of foods. I memorized food labels, analyzed the ingredient lists and religiously counted how many calories I ate each day. But I found the more I obsessed about the number of fat grams, carbs and calories I consumed, the more obsessed I was with eating altogether. When I tried to focus on eating right—cutting out butter, cream and mayo, eating lean meats and fish, avoiding an entire box of cookies or cake—maintaining my weight and even losing a few pounds became much easier.

I liken this scenario to that of someone who is out of work. Someone who doesn't have a job has a harder time finding one because he or she wants it so badly. The eagerness and obsession are all too evident to interviewers. Folks who have a job and financial security display an air of confidence that employers are seeking; and inevitably, these individuals are the ones who receive an offer.

The more you obsess with the calories in a piece of chicken or a bowl of cereal, the more eager you are to eat the food you're obsessing over. Willpower comes more easily when you concentrate more on maintaining good health and less on the weight you'd like to lose or food you can't have.

It's about changing habits, not analyzing every morsel of food you consume. If you eat more healthy food, more balanced meals and less junk, you won't even have to worry about calories, especially if you throw in a workout every now and then.

That being said, there are other good reasons to read food labels. If a label suggests there's more sugar, corn syrup, salt, preservatives and additives than nutritious ingredients, there's a good chance you shouldn't be eating whatever's in the package, regardless of calorie count.

I realize that lots of people have great success with the calorie-counting approach. If you're one of them, I give you great credit. If it DOES work for you, then by all means keep doing it. Better habits, moderation and balance have worked better for me. Not to mention, between P&L's, tax returns and research reports, I've got way too many calculations running through my head as it is.

# DON'T SKIP MEALS

Many people think they'll lose weight by cutting out breakfast or lunch, thus omitting a vast number of calories from their daily intake. However, less isn't always a better idea.

I went down this track in college, thinking if I skipped a meal, my stomach would shrink and I'd desire less food in subsequent meals. What happened instead was I'd obsess about food during the hours until my next meal. Then I'd devour way too much food, because I was truly hungry by the time I actually ate. If edible packaging had been available 25 years ago, I probably would have eaten my plate, too. Skipping meals only makes you eat more in the long run.

Though this is an opinion I feel passionately about, the scientific data is mixed. Fasting in a controlled diet environment can have weight-loss benefits for obese individuals. But this book is not for individuals with serious health issues such as obesity or diabetes. If you are only 10-15 pounds overweight or close to an ideal weight and simply too busy to eat, skipping meals can unfavorably impact your health.

When you skip a meal (or two or three), your body starts to wonder why it's not getting any food and goes into starvation mode, thus slowing down your metabolism. If your metabolism slows down, you'll have a harder time burning whatever calories you do consume. And this is exactly the opposite of the effect you wanted when you cut out calories in the first place. A research study published in December 2007 in the *Metabolism* medical journal concluded that skipping meals during the day and eating one large meal in the evening resulted in potentially risky metabolic changes. Elevated fasting glucose levels and delayed insulin responses can lead to diabetes over time.

I'm one of those lucky individuals diagnosed with Irritable Bowel Syndrome. After years of malicious stomach pains (ones I still sometimes have), I had every test in the universe to make sure there wasn't something horribly wrong with me. I am convinced that, with any stomach or intestinal ailment, the diagnosis "IBS" really stands for "I Bet it's Something, but don't know what."

To alleviate my symptoms, in addition to recommended dietary alterations, my doctor suggested I try eating more meals each day. The hope was that adding a snack in the morning and again in the afternoon might relax my system enough to reduce my aches and pains. I followed her advice and thought for sure I'd gain weight. I felt like all I was eating food incessantly; and in fact, at one point I actually got tired of eating (the first time in my life I could say that!). The net result of switching to five meals a day was no weight gain at all. I'm not sure if I ate less at my "big" meal-time, or if my body's fuel supply was so consistent that my metabolism picked up.

Consistency is key, because your metabolism adapts to your body's current weight. The last thing you want to do is skip meals and throw everything out of whack. Another downside to skipping meals? When you're starving, you're much more likely to dive into a bag of Tostitos or Kettle Chips. After all, binges tend to happen when your blood sugar is low and your need for sustenance is high. Those cravings are much easier to control when your stomach's not doing a song and dance.

# ESPECIALLY NOT BREAKFAST

Though I have already professed the value in not skipping meals, breakfast deserves its own mention. There are three things which are known to influence a person's metabolic rate: exercise, strength training and eating breakfast. Your body is somewhat deprived of nutrients after a good night of sleep, and your metabolism has **slowed down as well**. Breakfast picks it back up again! If you miss morning nutrients, your body will start the day in an energy lull, which can negatively affect your alertness and concentration. If you mask that hunger with three cups of coffee, you'll only exacerbate the problem.

A breakfast high in protein tends to keep my belly much more full for the rest of the morning, helping prevent unhealthy snack attacks (like the day old donuts lying around in the break room). Eggs are a great source of protein, assuming your cholesterol level isn't exorbitantly high, and lean meats like ham and turkey can be a nice accompaniment. Though bacon and sausage are tasty, they contain saturated fat and possibly nitrates as well. Luckily, there are lots of great substitutes today, like turkey bacon or chicken sausage. Make sure you check the nutrition labels to ensure the "lean" substitutes are actually lower in fat and calories. And as always, keep moderation in mind.

My grandfather was always a big breakfast eater and now I laugh when I think of that big old bowl of oatmeal he ate each day. Though oatmeal is a nice choice for a morning meal, my "Nannanny" would put about ½ stick of butter and ¼ cup of sugar on top of his. This probably wasn't the ideal preparation for someone with heart disease (nor were the cigarettes he "hid" under the driver's seat in his car)!

My grand mom always made him home-made biscuits, too. And boy, were they good! I loved to watch her make them by placing two to three cups of self-rising flower in a big bowl. Then she'd carve a hole in the middle of the flour and fill it with buttermilk and a rather large dollop of Crisco. Next, she'd simply work her fingers from the inside out until the whole concoction was thoroughly mixed.

She rolled out the dough, cut individual biscuits and bake them at 350 degrees for about 12–15 minutes. As if the Crisco wasn't enough, one simply *had* to add more butter to the biscuits as soon as they came out of the oven. I still make these on special occasions, but I try to cut back the amount of fat I use. I can't believe my grand mom went to the trouble to make these every day.

Another great southern accompaniment to almost any breakfast dish, but especially eggs, is grits. I know a lot of folks roll their eyes and say "YUK!" when they hear the word grits (the same people that eat polenta at night time and claim to be very sophisticated, even though the two are essentially the same).

The secret to making good grits is NOT to make them with water only. By substituting milk for water, or at least a milk/water mixture, you give the grits a completely different, creamier consistency. It's important to add salt while you're cooking them, too, so the flavor isn't bland. And though butter adds wonderful flavor, you won't need much.

# Recipes
Breakfast is still a tradition in our household, so I'm including some of our favorites.

### The Egg Sandwich

> 2 slices whole-grain bread, buttered slightly and broiled in the oven (*I'm convinced bread is not as good in the toaster as it is broiled in the oven with a little butter or olive oil on it*)
> Roasted tomatoes (see page 31)
> Fried eggs (*the sandwich is much easier to eat if you cook the eggs until well done*)
> Cheese (*I really like a creamy cheese like Port Salut or havarti*)

Assemble the sandwich in layers with the cheese on top. Place it briefly under the broiler to melt the cheese. The secret is the roasted tomatoes, and it tastes sensational.

## The Egg Bagel

I had the best one of these I ever tasted at a bagel shop in Vancouver, BC, on our way from Seattle to Whistler for another glorious weekend of skiing.

> Toasted bagel (*fresh from the bagel shop tastes best*)
> Cream cheese
> Chives or green onions
> Fresh parsley
> Canadian bacon, cooked (*substitute with turkey bacon or prosciutto if preferred*)
> Fried egg, cooked thoroughly
> Chopped onion
> Avocado, sliced
> Salsa

Compile cream cheese with green onions and parsley. Spread on toasted bagel. Pile remaining ingredients on top. It's heavenly, and a little twist on the usual egg sandwich.


## Homemade Granola

Friends and family have told me I should start a business selling this stuff. But I use the recipe to make holiday gifts instead. Store-bought brands do not hold a candle to the taste of this golden, delicious cereal, inspired by a recipe from Ina Garten. I like mine served with plain yogurt. Though the recipe makes 12 cups, I usually double it due to popular demand.

> 4 cups rolled oats
> 2 cups sweetened, shredded coconut (*unsweetened is not as good*)
> 2 cups sliced almonds
> ¾ cup canola oil
> ½ cup honey
> 1 cup golden raisins
> 1 cup dried cranberries
> 1 cup cashews

1. Preheat oven to 325 degrees.
2. Mix the oats, coconut and almonds in a large bowl.

3. Whisk together the oil and honey (*sometimes I heat the honey in a microwave for about 20 seconds so it mixes more easily*). Pour the liquids over the oat mixture and stir until nuts and oats are coated.

4. Pour onto large baking sheet. Bake, stirring every 15 minutes (*a bit more often near the end*), until golden brown, usually about 45-50 minutes in total. The secret is the cooking! As it nears the end of baking, it cooks exponentially faster. If you cook it too long, it gets dry. I like it best just as it's turning a deep gold color.

5. Remove the granola from oven and allow it to cool, stirring occasionally (*otherwise you'll have a big block of granola that's near impossible to break apart*).

6. Add the fruit and cashews and store in airtight container. If you like another type of dried fruit better than cranberries or raisins, feel free to add it in place of or in addition to those that I suggest.

## Pancakes

On lazy weekend mornings, sometimes you have to cave and make some good old fashioned pancakes (or "pan pakes," as my son calls them). I know, they are an indulgence, but you just have to spoil and reward yourself with a morning sweet every now and then. And if you cut them up to look like Easter bunnies and creatively add eyes and mouths with edible items you have stored in your pantry, you child will eat them up!

My recipe feeds three to four people.

> 1 cup flour (*whole wheat flour improves the flavor, I think*)
> 1 tablespoon sugar
> ½ tsp salt
> ¾ teaspoon baking powder
> ½ teaspoon baking soda
> 1 egg
> 1 cup buttermilk (*or plain yogurt, with a little extra milk to thin out the batter*)
> 2 tablespoons melted butter

Mix the dry ingredients. Then mix the wet ingredients in a separate bowl. Combine and stir until just mixed. Add fresh fruit, bananas or walnuts to bring in a little nutritional value and flavor. Ladle onto a hot, greased surface, flip when bubbles appear, and cook until browned on the bottom.

# WATCH WHAT YOU EAT OUT

It is often easy to "be good" when you cook at home. You can control the grocery list, food portions, recipe selection and amount of butter you add. It's a little harder when you visit a local restaurant for a meal out. One never knows just what has been added to make those vegetables taste so much better than when you have steamed them at home.

Though I like to cook at home, it's a treat to discover the culinary creations of others, be waited upon and not have to clean a kitchen. And if you travel for work or pleasure, you will have to deal with eating at restaurants, at the airport or on a plane, if food is actually served.

I have Five Restaurant Commandments to which I *try* to adhere in keeping the calorie count under control. These allow you to eat well without feeling like a greasy blob the next time you are sitting in business meeting after a big lunch or collapse onto the couch after a long, hard day of work.

## 1. Stay away from creamy sauces.

Whether you are at a fine Italian restaurant or visiting the local pub, pick the dishes with redder sauces. White sauces consist of butter and cream, any way you sauté it, and that spells a fattening combination that's not good for you. There are certainly lighter white sauces consisting primarily of wine or lemon, with a touch of cream; and I find these delicious and healthy to eat. Generally speaking, though, you tend to see this type of sauce at a higher-end establishment. If you aren't sure how much cream a dish might contain, just ask your server; he'll be happy to tell you. If their response is "It's filling" or "It's pretty rich," I recommend deferring.

Red sauces, such as marinara, rarely have cream and butter, unless it's a vodka sauce or one called out as a tomato cream sauce. Tomato-based sauces are generally seasoned with a little olive oil, garlic and other seasonings. And this spells a healthy, low-calorie dish that tastes good, too.

So if the choice is red or white, pick red.

## 2.  Watch the appetizer selection.

Unfortunately, most appetizers on any menu are fattening. Half of them are fried, ranging from fried mushrooms to fried calamari to fried chicken wings. The other class of appetizers are ones laden with cheese, including nachos, quesadillas and fried cheese (the double whammy).

Appetizer selections can also be heavy on the mayonnaise, such as the artichoke parmesan selection. And don't let veggies in the name fool you. They can be masked by lots of other unhealthy and fattening ingredients.

Even tossed salads, if loaded down with blue cheese or ranch dressing, aren't necessarily a healthy choice. Again, salads vary by restaurant. Some arrive with an army of ham, bacon bits and cheese; others are topped with apples and walnuts. Some swim in an ocean of dressing; others are lightly tossed. If you order dressing on the side, you can more easily limit your intake. But blue cheese and other mayonnaise-based dressings will be fattening no matter how little you use.

## 3.  Don't order French fries.

I know. It's hard for me, too. But if you don't order them, you don't eat them. Or you can steal a fry or two off your spouse's plate and satisfy your yearning without ingesting an entire serving of grease. So when you have a choice of fries, dig down deep and say no. You'll feel better afterwards for exhibiting French fry willpower.

## 4.  Watch your appetite after multiple glasses of wine.

I, for one, find that my desire for food intensifies with each glass of wine. Wine usually enhances the flavor food, so the more you drink, the more you want to eat. I'm not suggesting you turn away a glass or two of wine, especially if you are eating at a restaurant with an extensive selection. Just be aware of how each additional glass can impair your eating judgment. Not only might you eat a larger quantity of food, but you may be tempted to order lower quality dishes as well.

## 5.   If you must have dessert, share it with someone else.

I absolutely love to order dessert at the end of a good meal, especially if bread pudding or key lime pie is on the menu. In fact, I have nearly gotten in fork fights over how much of the dessert I personally devour when I do share. But still, I eat less when I agree to dividing a dessert in two (even if my husband would question the size of my "half"). Even though I might want the entire piece or slice at the time, I'm perfectly full and satisfied with a smaller portion by the time I'm driving (or biking!) home.

Bon appétit!

# SPICE THINGS UP

Good food doesn't have to bland or boring, and sometimes all it takes is a little spice or an unexpected ingredient to make all the difference. Though my list continues to expand as I try more dishes and learn more from others, I'll include a few helpful hints and ideas to make even the most ho-hum dishes a little more interesting.

## Recipes

### Roasted Tomatoes
Do you like tomatoes as much as I do? Do you live for those fresh, sweet, luscious fruits that grow in your backyard during the summer? Are you sad when the first frost arrives and you must say goodbye to the last remaining green treasures you were hoping would turn to red? Store-bought winter tomatoes simply don't hold a candle to the real thing. Sometimes you can find sweet grape tomatoes that almost do the trick. But another great option you may not have tried is roasting tomatoes. They taste great on egg sandwiches, turkey sandwiches or pretty much anything in which you place the plump and luscious summer vegetable.

> Roma tomatoes, thinly sliced (about ¼")
> Salt, pepper
> Olive oil

1. Drizzle olive oil over tomatoes and season with salt and pepper. (*In the summer months, chop some fresh basil or oregano and sprinkle on the top.*)
2. Spread out on a baking sheet and bake for 15 minutes at 425 degrees.
3. Don't overcook them or they get a burned flavor. Leftovers last in the fridge for several days.

## Panini Sandwiches

I paid $30 for a Panini maker at Target, and it's one of the best purchases I have ever made (I have no idea why anyone needs to pay $100 or more for a high-end brand). Paninis simply taste better than cold sandwiches or those broiled in the oven, and I'm not sure why.

For the uninitiated, a Panini maker is like a waffle iron for sandwiches. It turns an ordinary sandwich into something special: hot and crusty on the outside and chewy, gooey on the inside. And whether you are making a ham or turkey sandwich, or perhaps an all-veggie tomato and mozzarella concoction, there's a secret ingredient to making them taste fabulous. We discovered this at a wonderful little restaurant in McCall, Idaho, called Bistro 45. You add a mixture of mayonnaise and pesto and it adds an incredible flavor. The restaurant recommended a 5:1 ratio of mayo:pesto. But we tend to veer towards a 1:1 mix to cut the fat, and also because we are addicted to basil!

## Basil Pesto

This is a slight variation on a recipe found in the Moosewood Restaurant cookbook. Not only is it great on sandwiches, but it tastes wonderful with pasta and fish as well.

> 2½ cups firmly packed fresh basil leaves
> 2 large garlic cloves, chopped
> ½ cup pine nuts, walnuts or almonds
> ½ cup freshly grated Parmesan cheese (*I usually use a bit more and strongly prefer a high-quality, Italian Parmesan cheese*)
> ½ cup olive oil
> Lemon to taste
> Salt to taste

Mix the dry ingredients in a food processor then add the olive oil in a slow, steady stream until a smooth paste is formed. The pesto will last for several weeks, and the lemon juice helps prevent discoloration.

## Sweet Potato Fries

Once you start making sweet potato fries, you'll never want fries made with Idaho Baking Potatoes again. I probably shouldn't say that since I live in Idaho, and since I sometimes fire up a combination of the two. Either way, you can chop the peeled sweet potatoes like standard fries or cube them. I have even used my mandolin to create thin, chip-like slices (this version doesn't have to be cooked as long, however). It really doesn't matter because they taste fabulous any ole way.

After spreading the pieces out across a baking sheet, being careful not to pile too many on top of one another, pour on the olive oil to ensure all the potatoes are coated. You can also season them with salt, pepper and fresh rosemary, or even chili powder, red pepper, coriander and/or oregano. I tend to use whatever I have in my house or select seasonings to complement whatever else I happen to be cooking that night.

Bake them in a hot oven (around 425 degrees), being careful not to burn them. Depending on how thick the slices are, they may stay in the oven for 30–45 minutes, with a "stir" halfway in between.

## Arugula Salad

Arugula is something I discovered recently, now that it's more readily available in standard grocery retailers, though I have grown it quite abundantly in my own garden as well. This green has a more bitter taste than standard lettuces, so it holds the flavor of lemon or vinegar better. The stark flavor contrasts with other dishes you prepare, and really adds a boost to the meal. I like to keep arugula salad simple—adding only avocado, tomato and very thin slices of red onion. I then make a dressing of salt and pepper, olive oil and fresh lemon juice. After you've mixed it together, give it a taste. If it's not lemony enough, squeeze in a little more.

For a different twist, you can add goat cheese, toasted almonds and dried cranberries (and fresh herbs if you have them available). I tend to like a dressing of olive oil and balsamic vinegar with these ingredients.

Arugula is wonderful. So next time you buy greens, try it out!

## Baked Broccoli

I have always liked steamed broccoli with a little lemon and olive oil, but recently a friend of mine from my former Seattle Running Club (also known as the Wining Women) introduced me to the delights of baked broccoli. To make this new take on an old veggie, simply chop the broccoli into bite-sized pieces and spread across a baking sheet. Then drizzle with olive oil and sprinkle with steak seasoning and garlic powder. Bake the broccoli for 15 minutes at 425 degrees. If it's a little crisp, it's even better.

## Sliced Brussels Sprouts

As much as I like Brussels sprouts, I couldn't for the life of me get my family to eat them until I tried cooking them up in disguise one night. My magic act worked! Thinly slice the Brussels sprouts (after you have pulled off the outer bitter edges) as if you are slicing cabbage. Place in a pan and add about a tablespoon of olive oil. From there, you can add what you like—my favorite seasonings are garlic and capers. You can also add sliced shallots, red pepper flakes or even pancetta. Sauté the Brussels sprouts about 10–15 minutes over medium-low heat. Feel free to taste-test to make sure they don't get mushy.

## Grilled Vidalia Onions

I have tried many varieties of sweet onions, such as Walla Wallas, but none of them compare to the Vidalia onions grown in Toombs County, Georgia. Besides, how many vegetables have a museum named after them? Though they are available late-April until mid-November, here in the Northwest I can only seem to find them in the early summer. When grilled, they taste wonderful atop a steak or burger, but they are also good by themselves or combined with other fresh, grilled veggies. Here's how I prepare them:

1. Slice about ¼" thick and douse with olive oil.
2. Season with salt and pepper and cook on a hot grill for about 10 minutes, flipping once.

Vidalia onions are also good source of vitamin C and dietary fiber. So what are you waiting for?

**Turkey Burgers, Turkey Chili, Turkey Tacos….Just Use Turkey**
I rarely use ground beef anymore, because ground turkey is so much leaner and better for you and the difference in taste is hardly noticeable. I just substitute ground turkey in any dish that calls for ground beef without any other ingredient substitution or alteration.

The only exception to that is the classic burger, when you're eating the meat "straight" rather than camouflaged in a sauce or mixture. Because turkey is not as naturally flavorful as beef or buffalo, I like to spice up the patties with chili powder, paprika, and even onion powder and garlic powder. And of course salt and pepper. They taste wonderful when grilled or broiled.

**Tuna with a Kick**
I realize that, thanks to the mayo, tuna salad sandwiches are not exactly the healthiest things you can eat, but I have loved them since I was a little girl. They were also my "pickles and ice-cream" during pregnancy. Using tuna canned in water and adding mayonnaise sparingly, it's not *too* horrible for you. Recently, I discovered a wonderful tuna melt at a local coffee shop called Java. They told me the secret to their tuna salad was dill and cayenne pepper. I have made it at home with a generous helping of those two spices, also adding some chopped red onion and salt, and it's as good as the café's. When you top the tuna with roasted tomatoes and a nice slice of low-fat cheese and broil it in the oven, it's even better.

## Brown Rice with Fruit and Nuts

To make white rice, the bran layer from brown rice is removed in the milling process, and along with it go nutrients like vitamin E, thiamin, riboflavin, niacin, vitamin B6, folacin, potassium, magnesium, iron and more than a dozen others. Based on its nutritional makeup, why don't we all eat brown rice? Perhaps because our taste buds have adapted to white race if that's what we have eaten most of our lives.

Sauces and broths can help transition your palette to the wilder flavor of brown rice. The following recipe is based on one I found in *Cuisine at Home Magazine*, modified with my own touches. The result is anything but bland and complements a number of entrees as a side dish. It serves four.

> ½ cup brown rice
> ¾ cup water
> ¾ cup chicken broth
> ¼ cup chopped onion (*I sometimes add a little more*)
> 1 tablespoon olive oil
> ½ teaspoon cinnamon
> ¼ cup dried cherries or cranberries
> ¼ cup nuts (*pecans, sliced/slivered almonds, or walnuts*)

1. Sauté the chopped onion in olive oil for two to three minutes with the cinnamon.
2. Add the rice and cook a few minutes more, stirring.
3. Add the liquids and simmer for about 45 minutes.
4. When the rice has absorbed most of the liquids, add the fruit and nuts. Let it sit about another five minutes and then serve.

# BEWARE OF APPETIZERS

As I've mentioned earlier, skipping meals can impair your eating judgment. When your stomach is empty and energy is low, you are more susceptible to scarfing down unhealthy treats to satisfy your hunger.

Even if you're not starving, snack time can be danger time, especially before dinner. If you fill up on snacks, you're less likely to eat a healthy, nutrient-rich main course. It's easy to nibble while you're cooking or even watching someone else prepare a meal (especially when it's my husband, who is known for wonderful meals that take HOURS to prepare). So be vigilant! If you must snack to stave off your hunger, be wary of the fat-rich, nutrient-deprived treats.

## The Ones to Watch Out For

### Chips and Salsa

My husband can down half a bag of Tostitos in less than five minutes, and he does so with regularity before dinner. I constantly remind him, when he complains about his love handles, that he's getting lots of love from fried corn. Chips, consisting of a vegetable which is comparatively lower in nutrients in the first place, are stripped of anything healthy during processing and then deep fried to add that proverbial icing on the cake.

No matter how good they taste and how harmless they may seem, tortilla chips are not a great way to fill your belly. Even if the salsa is fresh and full of veggies.

### Cheese and Crackers

Crackers may not be that horribly bad for you—at least the ones that aren't deep fried—but there's nothing of benefit in them for you either. Let's take a look at saltines. Here's the ingredient list: *enriched flour, riboflavin, folic acid, soybean oil and/or partially hydrogenated cottonseed oil, high-fructose corn syrup, salt leaving, malted barley flour.*

Not very reassuring, is it? And though cheese has nutritional value as I've already discussed, those triple-cream brie cheeses can pack in the fat. Even if they do taste darn good!

## French Onion Dip with Chips

You've likely eaten French onion dip or made it at some point in your life, if for no other reason than because of how quick and easy it is to assemble. It pleases the palate and satisfies guests, keeps the pocketbook happy and can be thrown together in minutes. But it consists of highly processed soup mix and at least two cups of sour cream. Need I say more?

Adding to the bad news is the fact that we scoop this stuff up with potato chips, fried in oil and heavily salted. Not exactly a nutritionist's dream.

## Artichoke Dip

Have you ever wondered what was in baked artichoke dip? It's always a real crowd pleaser, but when I pull out my mom's recipe, I see how it's made and why it tastes so good:

> 1 can of artichoke hearts, chopped
> 1 cup mayonnaise
> 1 cup parmesan cheese
> ½ teaspoon garlic salt
> 1 tablespoon lemon juice

After cooking for 20 minutes at 350 degrees, (sadly) a thin layer of grease forms on the top. And you can't exactly scoop up the dip by the spoonful (well, I guess you could), so you'll need to eat it with some sort of not-so-healthy chip or cracker. By the time all is said and done, you feel as if you're harming guests who consume it with a special artery-clogging formula. Who wants to be guilty of that?

## Chicken Wings

Save face and don't say grace before this snack. However you like to spice 'em up, with honey mustard, barbeque sauce or garlic and ginger, this dish needs to be on its way out of your repertoire. Hooters may have made them famous, but now Foster Farms makes them easy to serve straight from your oven. Don't go there.

## Healthier Alternatives

Raw vegetables, as boring as they may be, are a great alternative to chips, dips and wings. Especially if you don't pour an entire bottle of ranch or blue cheese dressing on top. If I'm at someone else's house for a dinner party, I MAKE myself eat the veggies, because it's almost impossible to consume too much dressing without re-creating a *Seinfeld* episode by double dipping.

My husband likes to chop a big variety of veggies at the start of the week to store in a Tupperware container. Then whenever he is starving, he dives into something healthy (assuming the Tostitos have already vanished). This is a great way to make it easier to choose a healthy alternative.

There are other great, healthy appetizers as well. Check them out!

## Recipes

### Steamed Artichokes

Steamed artichokes are a wonderful appetizer, and are hearty enough to pinch-hit as a main course. I steam mine for about 30 minutes unless it's a gigantic one like you find in California. Admittedly, it's hard to eat an artichoke without some sort of dipping sauce, and I am particularly partial to a garlic aioli. You'll consume less mayonnaise with your veggie for fear of what it might do to your breath the next day, despite its wonderful taste.

> ½ cup mayonnaise
> 2–3 garlic cloves, chopped finely
> 1–2 teaspoons of lemon, to taste
> Freshly ground black pepper
>
> Mix it together and it's good to go!

## Brushetta

This is wonderful appetizer to make, especially in the summer when you can select fresh, delicious tomatoes from your own garden. All you have to do is chop tomatoes and add balsamic vinegar and olive oil, plus fresh basil. Add a little salt and pepper, then spoon over slices of fresh whole-grain bread. It's an absolutely wonderful snack that carries some nutritional value as well.

## Tomato and Mozzarella Salad

This is not much different than bruschetta; just add a little cheese and skip the bread. It's fabulous and easy to make and, like its counterpart above, is much better in the summer when everything is fresh and flavorful.

## Fruit Smoothie

Another snack I enjoy and actually relish prior to a workout (rather than prior to a meal) is a fruit smoothie. This is the perfect snack for someone who struggles to eat fresh apples. And it's a great way to get some easily digested energy before a run or walk. Even kids love it.

> ½–¾ cup frozen or fresh fruit (*I use a frozen fruit medley with lots of berries*)
>
> ½ banana (*I honestly think a smoothie just doesn't taste right without a banana to thicken it up*)
>
> ½ cup soy milk (*tastes richer than lowfat cow's milk*)
>
> A scoop of protein powder
>
> Some ice if the fruit is fresh and not frozen

Other optional ingredients include plain yogurt, flax seeds, nuts (walnuts or almonds) or even juice if you like yours a little sweeter. A high-quality blender is a must.

# EAT MEAT OR NOT

I recently had the pleasure of carrying out market research to understand the cooking and shopping habits of moms, across an array of ages, income and expertise. The research, in particular, was to assess opinions and perceptions of meats, including pork, chicken and beef. (We did not interview vegetarians or vegans.) We actually went into the homes of these women, looking at their pantries, refrigerators and eating areas.

What I personally found most interesting was the inconsistency in perceptions about which type of meat is the healthiest. For some, it was clearly chicken; for others it was beef. A few felt that pork was the least healthy alternative because of the fattiness of pork chops. Another felt the slaughtering of chickens was so inhumane that she often avoided eating the bird altogether. A few ladies were unaware of how different cuts of meat each yielded a unique fat and health profile, not understanding the numbering system on ground beef labels.

I'm sure if we had interviewed non-meat eaters or fish-only eaters, we would have found an even broader range of conflicting feedback, opinions and perceptions.

For much of my life, especially after I lost that college weight, people have assumed I am vegetarian. I suppose this is because I am a healthy eater and the stereotype is that healthy eaters don't eat meat.

Speaking purely from a health perspective, even without addressing the less-than-optimal way animals are often treated, there are advantages of eliminating meat from your diet. Among them are a decreased chance of being overweight (unless you overdo the cheeses and dessert!). You'll be likely to consume more fiber and have a decreased risk of medical conditions such as colon cancer. You may even find yourself with more energy and a clearer complexion.

There are disadvantages, however. If you are vegetarian, you will probably consume less protein, which has important benefits. You'll likely intake less creatinine, which helps build muscle mass. You may even consume fewer vitamins and minerals in their natural form, especially if you are vegan.

Though I am in no way insisting that anyone convert to vegetarianism or, alternatively, become a lifelong Atkins Diet enthusiast, I do support the notion of moderation and paying careful attention to those meats you are eating, if you choose to eat them.

And though I couldn't begin to debate this topic in a two-page chapter, I thought I'd at least include a few thoughts on a healthier approach to eating meats.

**The other white meat**: Though many people assume that pork is too fatty to be healthy, a study by the USDA, University of Wisconsin and University of Maryland found that a 3 oz. (85 g) serving of pork tenderloin contains 0.105 oz. (2.98 g) of fat and that the same portion of skinless chicken breast contains 0.106 oz (3.03 g) of fat. On the downside, pork is lower than most cuts of beef in vitamin B-12, zinc and iron. Also, fatty, processed cuts, such as bacon and sausage, are high in saturated fats and may contain nitrates, which have been linked to cancer.

**The original white meat:** Chicken is high in protein and often less expensive than beef (unless you are buying ground beef or another inexpensive, and often fatty, cut). It's also low in fat if you cut off the skin before cooking. Chicken can be prepared in a great variety of ways, but baking, broiling, grilling and roasting tend to be the healthiest. Keep in mind that chicken needs to be well cooked to avoid any nasty bacteria. And fried chicken just doesn't cut it, no matter how you slice it or grease it up. Especially since there are nice alternatives these days, such as baked chicken with Corn Flakes.

**Fish**: Many types of fish—especially salmon and tuna—are packed with beneficial omega-3 fatty acids, which have been linked to decreased rates of heart disease. It is also believed that omega-3 fatty acids decrease triglycerides, lower blood pressure, reduce blood clotting, enhance immune function, improve arthritis symptoms and improve learning ability in children. According to the Mayo Clinic, fish may also lower your cholesterol by substituting unsaturated fatty acids for saturated fatty acids such as those found in meat. Though there are risks associated with the consumption of mercury, most research suggests that the benefits of consuming omega-3 fatty acids far outweigh them.

**Buffalo**: Buffalo is a great alternative to beef. It has much less fat and is typically grass-fed, making it easier on the environment as well as your arteries.

**Beef**: Grass-fed, pasture-raised cattle produce the highest quality meat, even more so than organic meats, because organic meat may be produced from cows that eat grain. Thanks to grazing in a more natural environment, grass-fed cattle grow more normally than those in factory farms or contained animal feeding operations (CAFOs).

As far as lean versus fat beef, "select" is the leanest cut you can buy, containing around 7 percent fat by weight. "Choice" contains 15 to 35 percent fat by weight. "Prime" is the fattiest grade, containing 35 to 45 percent fat by weight. Lean beef and veal cuts have the words "loin" or "round" in their names. Lean pork cuts have the words "loin" or "leg" in their names.

**Preparation**: Baking, broiling, grilling and roasting are the healthiest ways to prepare meat. For fish, poaching is also a great option. And it's always important, regardless of the type of meat you're eating, to cut out the visible fat before cooking.

# TREAT YOURSELF (ON OCCASION)

Not only do I like to sample sweets at restaurants, I pretty much like to eat sweets all the time. Baking up treats was my way of entertaining friends during high school and making cookies is a great source of entertainment for my little one when Dad's out of town. Of course, I still believe the best desserts on earth are made in the South. I'm not sure if it's the technique or the extra stick of butter that does the trick.

My love of sweets has been passed along from generation to generation in my family. When my mom shared her collection of our family's cherished childhood recipes, about half the book was filled with recipes for dessert. Even "green salads" were made with cups of sugar!

During college, when I gained all that weight, I decided the best way to remove some pounds was to eliminate sweets. Of course, the very thought of omitting sweets from my diet fueled my desire to have them that much more. So I'd go a few days without a morsel of chocolate or ice cream, and all of a sudden I would eat a package of cookies. And I'm not talking about a single serving package of cookies at the grocery checkout counter. I would make an entire box of Duncan Hines chocolate chip cookies and eat the whole batch. I'm not sure how I managed to do that without getting sick, but I remember having a sugar hangover the next day that was every bit as bad as the ones caused by alcohol. I know now how horribly I was treating my body by devouring sweets in such a huge quantity (talk about an insulin rush!).

Today, I eat sweets in moderation, cutting myself some slack. I try not to eat them every day; but when I do, I eat a piece of pie instead of the whole pie. Or a cup of ice-cream instead of a pint. And most importantly, a few cookies instead of the whole box.

I also have a few tricks that help ensure such moderation. When I make home-made chocolate chip cookies, I share the batter (it takes discipline!) and only cook a handful of cookies. Everyone gets one hot cookie and the rest of the dough goes in the freezer. I find that cooking them sparingly not only reduces the amount we'll eat in one sitting, it also means the cookies we do eat are freshly baked, and cookies taste so much better right out of the oven.

Another trick of mine is reducing the amount of sugar and/or butter in a recipe or substituting whole wheat for all-purpose flour. As with recipes from an earlier chapter, cutting back a little here and there usually saves fat and calories without much sacrifice in flavor. Baking can be tricky, though, and I admit you will sometimes end up with a flop on your hands when you experiment. I'm still a little leery about using sugar substitutes, but if sugar-free sweets help you curb your cravings, then stay with what works.

## Recipes

When you can tell a recipe has LOTS of something you shouldn't have, try cutting back on those ingredients. As you keep reducing the richness of recipes, pretty soon you'll find yourself unable to eat as many super-heavy foods as you once did. Now that's progress!

### Mom's Pumpkin Bread

Take my mom's pumpkin bread for example. She bakes this each year for Christmas presents, getting rave reviews from lucky recipients. My modifications are in italics.

> 1 No. 2 can pumpkin or pumpkin pie filling
> 3 cups sugar (*cut it to 2 cups*)
> 1 cup vegetable or canola oil (*try ½–¾ cup*)
> 4 eggs
> 1 teaspoon salt
> 1 heaping teaspoon cinnamon
> 1 teaspoon nutmeg
> 1 cup water
> 2 teaspoons soda
> 3½ cups all purpose flour (*experiment with whole wheat*)

1. Preheat oven to 350 degrees.
2. Mix all dry ingredients together.

3. Add remaining ingredients and mix well.
4. Coat pans with cooking spray and fill about two-thirds full.
5. Bake 45 minutes to one hour.

> Will make:    two 2 lb. sized pans
> four 1 lb. sized pans
> seven small loaf pans

## Hearty, Whole Wheat Chocolate Chip Cookies

You are going to be pleasantly surprised when you bit into these! I haven't removed any calories.

> ¾ cup granulated sugar
> ¾ cup brown sugar
> 1 cup butter, softened
> 1 teaspoon vanilla
> 2 eggs
> 2¼ cups whole wheat flour
> 1 teaspoon baking soda
> 1 teaspoon salt
> 1 bag milk chocolate chips

1. Heat oven to 350 degrees. In a large bowl, stir sugars, butter, vanilla and egg until well blended. Stir in flour, baking soda and salt. Add the chips last.
2. On ungreased cookie sheet, drop by rounded tablespoonfuls several inches apart.
3. Bake 8 to 10 minutes or until light brown.

## Caramel Cake

I originally got this recipe from *Cooking Light* and have made minor modifications so I don't have to buy special ingredients at the store before I make it. It has been a family and friend favorite for years. Though there's certainly no shortfall in sugar, the fat content of a typical cake has been reduced.

**Cake:**

>1½ cups granulated sugar
>½ cup butter, softened
>2 large eggs
>2¼ cups all-purpose flour
>2½ teaspoons baking powder
>1 teaspoon salt
>1½ cup fat-free milk
>2 teaspoons vanilla

1. To prepare cake, beat granulated sugar and butter at medium speed until well blended. Add eggs one at a time. Combine dry ingredients then add to sugar mixture, alternating with milk. Stir in vanilla.
2. Prepare pan(s) with cooking spray and dust with flour. Add batter, then cook at 350 degrees for about 30 minutes, until knife comes out clean in center of pans. Alter cooking time if using an especially deep pan. Cool.

**Frosting:**

>1 1/3 cups packed brown sugar
>½ cup milk (*nonfat works great*)
>¼ teaspoon salt
>3 tablespoons butter
>1 teaspoon vanilla
>2½–3 cups sugar

1. In a saucepan, combine brown sugar, milk and salt. Bring to a boil and reduce heat. Cook about five minutes or until slightly thickened.
2. Remove from heat; add butter and vanilla. Cool slightly.
3. Add powdered sugar and beat until smooth. I like to add the powdered sugar slowly to make sure icing doesn't get so thick you can't spread it out.
4. Spread icing evenly on top of cake. If preparing a layered cake, apply icing in between and all around.

# Shape Up!

Well I was born to run
To get ahead of the rest
And all that I wanted was to be the best
Just to feel free and be someone
I was born to be fast I was born to run

Emmylou Harris, "Born to Run"

# MEASURE YOUR FITNESS

There are five components to physical fitness commonly used by schools and health clubs as a testing measure.

1. **Cardiovascular endurance** is the ability of the heart and lungs to work together to provide the needed oxygen and fuel your body needs during sustained activity. To build cardiovascular endurance (a topic you'll be hearing a lot more about in subsequent chapters), you can run, cycle, cross-country ski, play basketball and numerous other activities.

2. **Muscular strength** is the ability of your body's muscle to generate force in a short period of time. In simpler terms, it's the amount of weight you can lift. You can build muscular strength by using exercises that involve lifting free weights, machine weights, or even your own body weight.

3. **Muscular endurance** measures how long you can work a particular set of muscles. To improve your muscular endurance, cardiovascular activities like running and biking do the trick for your lower body. Push-ups can build the endurance of your upper-body muscles.

4. **Flexibility** is the ability of all of the joints in the body to move through the full range of motion for each particular joint. Pilates and yoga are wonderful for improving flexibility, along with more basic stretching exercises.

5. **Body composition** is the ratio of fat mass to lean muscle mass, bone and organs. If you have an unusually high proportion of fat, you may be prone to illnesses or disease. Of course, it is humanly possible to have too much muscle mass, but it would take an excessive amount of lifting and dieting to get there.

Ideally, you should try to incorporate all five of these components into your workout routine. If you can run a marathon but cannot lift your three-month-old child, how balanced can your health possibly be? Likewise, a body builder who can't ride a bike for longer than five minutes may not be as physically fit as he or she thinks.

My thoughts on fitness are by no means as exhaustive and precise as those of a trained professional. Most of what I divulge I have learned the hard way, by experimenting, goofing up or healing aches and pains. Hopefully, these suggestions will help spare you some of my mistakes (and stubbornness).

If you work with a trained professional and get these components of your fitness tested, you will have a more precise idea of how to create your own personal fitness equation, including body parts to strengthen and/or improve. You probably have some idea of the kind of shape you're in already, but it never hurts to measure your fitness, so you can tailor a program to keep your body fit, firm, balanced and flexible.

# FIND SOMETHING
# THAT WORKS FOR YOU

When I was in the seventh grade, I attempted to play softball. And clearly the stars were not aligned for me to be a champion at this sport. Left field was always saved for the really bad players, so guess where they stuck me? Yep! Right out there where I could daydream the innings away. Whenever a fly ball finally did come my way, my mind was nowhere near the ballgame. I only lasted one season and the team was not sad to see me go.

I also tried track and cross-country, which I could do pretty well when I weighed ninety-five pounds in the seventh grade. However, I nearly killed myself to break a six-minute mile, something a gifted runner could do with ease. Not only that, I was such a klutz, I couldn't even pass a baton in a mile relay without tripping the next runner and colliding embarrassingly onto the track. When I gained some post-puberty weight, my track career came to a quick halt.

My family couldn't afford private lessons or club memberships to pursue tennis, so even though I liked the sport, I threw in the towel on this one until later in my life.

This pretty much left me playing basketball, a sport I could play reasonably well despite a rough start. In the tenth grade, I made my debut at full-court basketball; prior to this time, Tennessee had only allowed girls to play in the half-court, meaning three (guards) played defense and three (forwards) played offense (after all, running up and down an entire court was far too strenuous for females!). Having only played defense in junior high school, I was so excited to get the ball for the first time on offense, I accidentally ran down the court in the wrong direction, scoring an easy bucket for the opposing team.

It's the memory of these experiences that makes it hard for me to see myself as athletic. Even though I have completed eleven marathons to date, whenever someone suggests I am a good athlete, I still think they are talking to the person sitting beside me.

My history suggests that if I can get this fit, anybody can. In other words:

**You can enjoy working out and get good at it.....**
**.....even if you are not a fast runner, a world-class gymnast or a star in the NBA!**

I'm not sure if I was playing the wrong sports early in my life, or if I gained better balance and coordination as I grew older, but I have found my own way with a little experimentation, a few missteps and more than one mountain bike crash.

Your body, balance and abilities may change over time as well, so don't give up, despite potential setbacks. I strongly recommend trying a variety of sports and fitness activities in many different settings until you find an enjoyable combination which suits your skills, interests and personal fitness equation. Though your choices may be influenced by where you live, its natural terrain and weather conditions, you may never discover hidden talents or passions if you don't try a variety of things. It's much easier to make exercise a habit if it's fun.

To give you some ideas, I'll describe some of my own experiences and experiments.

**A team sport to mix and mingle**. When I turned 25, out of the blue, I decided I was going to have a second try at tennis. I still couldn't afford lessons, but I bought a new racket and signed up for a USTA certified league in Charlotte, North Carolina. The first time I played a league match was the first tennis match of my life, and I survived. In fact, I even won most of my 3.0 level matches that season. To this day, though I'm no Chris Evert, I can still put a little English on the ball, win some matches and even run my husband around on the court a bit. More importantly, tennis has remained a really fun way to run, strengthen muscles and sweat. And since playing tennis means you're required to hit a ball back and forth with someone else, it's also a way to socialize, make new friends and even have someone else hold you accountable for working out.

**A solo adventure to enjoy nature and the warmth of summer.** I never rode a mountain bike until I was 31 and living in Boston. And in fact, my first time out on the trails was a complete disaster. I went out riding with my then-boyfriend and had too much pride to admit I didn't know what I was doing. So when he decided to ride across a series of boulders (and not the smooth kind you see in Utah), I took a deep breath and gave it my best shot.

No sooner had I traversed a few of them than I had slammed on my brakes, flipped over my handlebars and landed on my wrist atop one of the rough and ragged rocks. Though I ended up having to walk home dejectedly that day, it didn't stop me from trying again and again and again. I soon came to realize that bumps and bruises were simply a part of the sport and nearly impossible to avoid (the scars on my legs prove it!). This somewhat nerve-wracking adventure may not be for you for this reason alone. But if you have trails nearby, enjoy the woods and like the thrill of steep climbs, rocks and roots, mountain biking might just be your sport.

**An outdoor adventure with exposure to the elements.** As much as I get annoyed with frozen fingers and toes, there's something magical about downhill skiing. Picking a line down a field of moguls is such a thrill, especially when you can stay on top of your skis and avoid a face plant. Even if you prefer groomed runs, the experience of being outdoors, breathing the fresh air and carving some turns is still hard to beat.

Before we all got married, my friends and I made annual expeditions to our favorite western locations. Whether it was Aspen, Telluride or Crested Butte, we shared endless laughter, drank too much beer and burned lots of calories in our die-hard attempts to ski all day, every day. At the end of each adventurous week, we felt refreshed, in shape and even a little sun-baked, despite all the SPF potions and lotions.

**A solo experience with a rush of endorphins.** Running, to me, isn't as fun and social as skiing or tennis or biking. But it has to be the easiest type of exercise to fit into your schedule, whether you are single or married, with children or not, travelling for work or busy at home. It's an excellent way to release stress, get energized or see the sights of a new city. All you need is a good pair of running shoes. You don't have to worry about flat tires, finding a partner or paying $80 a day to do it.

Even if you don't enjoy the actual run itself, the feeling that comes afterwards can be enough to keep you motivated. And it's never too late to give it a try. My friend Christina had never run in her life; then at age 37, she decided she wanted to run a marathon. With dedication and a supportive cast from Team in Training, a program sponsored by the Leukemia & Lymphoma Society, she completed the 26-mile distance in Portland. And, just as mothers forget the pain of childbirth, she has already forgotten the trip to the hospital afterwards (caused by over-hydration) and is ready to try it again!

**A sport to close the deal**. Though I am a pathetic golfer, as my 20-year-old Betty Jameson Kmart blue light special clubs clearly demonstrate, I have played. And many men and women swear by the sport as a business asset. Not only does a good golf game impress your boss or help make a sale, it also stimulates the mind, gets the blood moving and even burns a few calories if you stay out of the carts. Though it may not be as rigorous as a bike ride or a jog, and does cut into a good portion of your day, playing golf is still better than sitting at home on the couch. And if you're at all competitive (like me), you won't be able to resist keeping at it until you actually start getting better.

These experiences barely scratch the surface of all the many ways you can seek enjoyable exercise. There's also basketball, soccer, hiking and walking. And don't forget Ultimate Frisbee, boot camp courses and kickboxing to kick off your cardio training.

To work on your flexibility, you may prefer yoga or Pilates to sitting on the floor and stretching. If you wish to build muscle mass, scaling up a climbing wall may be a nice alternative to lifting barbells at the gym (better yet, go climbing outdoors!).

You don't need me to list all the possibilities, but I do suggest you try a few things you have never tried before. Keep in mind your motivations and preferences: whether you like to be indoors or out, with friends or alone, sweating or meditating. You simply have to try. Because if you like it, you will be more committed to it—and more likely to make it a habit and integral part of your life.

Try and try again, even if you don't succeed at first. After all, a bruised body part or ego doesn't stay in the way for long.

# MIX IT UP

Variety is the spice of life, and mixing up your exercise routine can go a long way in making fitness more fun, habit-forming and effective.

When I tell people I run marathons, they naturally assume I run every day and clock lots of miles. To the contrary, when I *finally* qualified for the Boston marathon, my training program consisted of only three days of running each week. Each workout varied: one long run (13–20 miles), one moderate run (6–7 miles) and one day of speed work. On the "off" days, I'd lift weights, attend a yoga class, go for a bike ride, or play a tennis match, depending on the season.

The more diverse the mix, the less I got bored with the running and, in my opinion, the better I was able to thwart a potential injury. Another reason I varied my workouts is that running doesn't do much in the way of firming up the booty or flattening the tummy. The more I integrate activities that stretch and strengthen my muscles, the less I slip and sag.

For years I have tried to convince my mom to try a daily walk. She gets bored with it, her knees hurt, or the weather's bad. Though I give her a hard time, the truth of the matter is I get bored walking, too, unless I'm in the hills with my crazy dogs. I get impatient with seeing the sights of my neighborhood at a slow, tedious pace.

Nonetheless, I highly recommend you try walking, because walking is very good for you! Not only does it burn calories (and tire out your furry creatures, if you have them), but walking is far more kind to your knees than running. Like running, it's also easy to integrate into the day, regardless of your work schedule or family demands. You can even vary the route to make your walks more interesting. One day you might walk near your office during lunch hour. The next, walk near home after you get home from the office. Maybe you can even walk *to* work, if you live close by. Better yet, you can drive to a trail at a nearby park or hill for a little scenic stimulation. Walk around the airport if your flight is delayed or take a stroll at the mall if you are really out of choices. Variety can be a real motivator.

In fact, there are at least as many physical benefits to variety as there are mental benefits. If you run five miles, five days a week for a year, your body adjusts and becomes more efficient. That means it doesn't need to recruit as many muscles or burn as many calories to perform the same activity. While in some ways you might see this as a good thing (less pain, for instance), the bad news is that you're not burning as many calories or challenging your muscles as much.

Little tweaks to the routine can have a big impact in keeping your body less bored and more engaged. For example, if you are trying to firm up your biceps, you might alternate between free weights and a pulley bicep curl. Instead of running nine-minute miles for five miles every day, throw in a tempo run or a speed workout every few days, as I did with my marathon training.

And don't just stick to the activities we typically think of as "working out." As we age and our bodies become (sadly!) more susceptible to gravity, variety goes a long way toward toning and firming. Remember that a day of skiing or tennis can help tighten the tush, and substituting 60 minutes of yoga for lifting weights can still work your arms and tone those triceps.

So mix it up, and your body will appreciate it.

# FIND A GYM THAT SUITS YOUR STYLE

Do you enjoy the gym? Can you go there for days on end without getting bored or do you often feel like one more mile on the treadmill or one more step on the StairMaster may send you to the loony bin? Maybe you're one of those lucky kickboxing or aerobics superstars who can avoid the doldrums. Or maybe the following statements more accurately describe your feelings about the gym.

> "It's too boring."
> "I would rather be outside."
> "I get annoyed when men and women spend more time hitting on each other than working out."
> "I don't want someone of the opposite sex to see me in shorts."
> "I don't know how to use the machines and feel too embarrassed to ask."

Regardless of your sentiments, a gym is a great outlet for exercise. Gyms are a great escape when you need to get out of the house, especially if you work from a home office. And they almost always have a great selection of free weights and machines for strength building, something a workout room at home may lack.

When I was in college, just shortly after I'd gained that freshman 25, I decided I needed to do something to lose some weight. Even though I'd gotten back into the routine of running again, I still needed an alternative for those cold, wintry days in North Carolina (and I admit that my definition of "cold and wintry" is certainly relative). I couldn't bear the thought of a fellow (male) student seeing me at the university gym in my tights or shorts, despite the improbability of a coed even noticing me in the first place.

So I joined an all-women gym on the other side of to Chapel Hill. This was great, because no matter how I looked or felt, I didn't have to watch all those beautiful, skinny, Carolina gals flirting with handsome men. And I didn't have to think about what I wore or worry if a few bulges fell beneath my shorts when I bent over to lift the barbells. The drive across town had its perils, though. Ironically enough, I totaled my car that year because I was peering ever so desperately to check out the flavors of the day at TCBY on the way home from the all-girls gym!

The point is that my strategy worked. Instead of letting my self-consciousness keep me out of the gym, I found a way around it. Think about your own reasons for going or avoiding, and come up with your own solutions. If a coed gym is your preference, then find one that offers the amenities you enjoy in a health club, like climbing walls, basketball courts or personal trainers. And if you have a small child, a health club that offers child care can really save the day. Just don't take a two-month-old baby into the weight room like I tried to do once.

I happen to prefer my local YMCA because I feel like it's a little less intimidating, a lot less sales-y, and presumably not as pick-up-y as other health clubs or gyms in town. In addition, our Y does amazing things for the community and it's nice to support such an organization. If your town doesn't have a YMCA, there may be a similar facility that suits your style and follows a similar mission.

My other strong recommendation is to join a health club close to home. Making exercise part of your everyday routine is very much about convenience. If you have to add 30 minutes to your workout just to get to the gym and back, there's a much greater likelihood you'll avoid it altogether. The closer the better, especially on rainy, cold nights when it's hard to get yourself out the door in the first place (ahh... memories of Seattle winters).

When you're traveling on business and only have time to exercise when it's dark outside, hotel gyms can be a godsend. Most of them are well equipped and convenient these days.

Once you've gotten regular visits to the gym worked into your life, don't forget to apply the "mix it up" strategy. Someone asked me recently if she should walk on the treadmill or lift weights when she frequented the gym. My answer was a definite, "Both!" Not only do I feel strongly about strength conditioning, but even with cardio training, the more you can add variety to your daily routine, the more likely you'll avoid burnout.

Whether you alternate between StairMasters, exercise bikes or pools, or integrate an aerobics class into the routine, each activity conditions you in a beneficial way. Take advantage of yoga or Pilates classes if your gym includes them in the membership package. My gym offers summer spinning classes outdoors at 5:30 a.m., so folks can spin while watching the sun rise. What better way to start the day?

I have one last tidbit. If you are a sports fan like I am, I recommend jumping on a stationary bike and watching a good basketball or football game. Most gyms have some way for you to view the TV while you pedal, climb, jump or run; and nothing spurs a little adrenalin rush like 3-point shots or touchdowns by your favorite players or team. I realize an exercise purist might not need a TV or an iPod, but if this type of entertainment minimizes the pain and adds to the thrill, then go for it!

# MAKE EXERCISE A
# PART OF YOUR SCHEDULE

Whether it's eating well, exercising or getting your dog to sit down and stay, repetition is critical. That's right. Do it over and over until it becomes a habit (incorporating variety in exercise, of course). Do it so much that if you don't do it, you start to feel terrible. That's when you know a habit has genuinely become part of your routine.

My mother-in-law once asked me, "How do you manage to fit in your workouts every day? It always seems like you find a way, regardless of the time, place or schedule." She's right. I'm disciplined, at least in some aspects of my life. I was never a student who liked to cram a semester's worth of knowledge the night before the final.

But even if you are not the most disciplined creature by nature, you can learn to build habits by scheduling. For example, if you are training for a triathlon and you know you need to swim, bike and run at some point during a given week, it's good to think about when and where you'll be able to do each activity before the week begins. If you are travelling for business one day, it's not likely you'll be carrying your bike alongside the briefcase. So make that day your run. Likewise, it's hard to find pools in an unfamiliar city when you are busy fighting traffic and getting to a meeting promptly, so schedule the swim when you're back in town. If you have a meeting after work one day, get up early to exercise before the workday begins. Or sneak away during your lunch hour.

It works best if you actually write your schedule down at the start of the week. There's something about seeing a schedule in writing that promotes follow-through.

I really sit down and think through the whens, hows and whats at the start of the week. I recommend that you do the same, whether your exercise ritual starts on Saturday, Sunday or Monday. And I also allow myself a day off each week. Treating yourself to a "free day" is a nice reward for six days of workouts well done. Recovery is an important part of training, too, so it's good to give the ole body some rest, regardless of how old it is.

So, make exercise a habit by scheduling it each week. You'll be amazed at how bad you'll feel if you don't stick to the plan. And sometimes feeling bad is a great motivator to start taking action that makes you feel better.

# CHALLENGE YOURSELF

I am big proponent of athletic events and challenges; I'm guessing a competitive spirit does this to a person. Having now watched my son want to beat me in everything from riding bikes to playing Candy Land to walking down the stairs, I know I passed along this beloved competitive gene honestly. Even if your biggest competitor is yourself, athletic events and challenges add focus and incentive to the usual daily routine.

Take my in-laws as an example. My mother and father-in-law have purchased pedometers to track the steps they take during the day, whether they are climbing stairs, walking to a local market or hiking in the beautiful hills of Santa Fe. They compete against one another for daily bragging rights in a non-threatening way. And regardless of who wins, by wearing the instrument throughout the day and comparing notes in the evening, they are keeping exercise front and center in their lives.

So whether you are tracking your steps to out-pace your spouse or challenging a friend to see who can eat the fewest sweets in a week, a little friendly competition can go a long way toward helping you reach your health and fitness goals.

There is a dark side to being competitive, though. Overdoing it can lead to injury and/or anxiety. So I have a few cautionary suggestions.

## Don't Worry About Coming in Last

When I was running the 2009 Boston marathon, I saw a wonderful sign that someone was wearing on her back. It said, "Relax. Neither one of us is going to win." What a great mantra for anyone other than Kara Goucher or Dire Tune! It was a great message to remind all of us of the honor to participate in the world's oldest annual marathon—and finish. So enjoy the experience of your event, regardless of your final time.

A long time ago, not long after I'd learned to mountain bike, I decided to sign up for a race in New Hampshire. "It'll be fun!" I told myself. I had a partner in crime, was in decent shape and figured I had nothing to lose. Meanwhile, I bought a pair of clipless pedals which happened to arrive the night before the race (clipless pedals—or "clip-ins" —lock your cycling shoes to the bike pedal to maximize power transfer and efficiency). If you have ever used this type of pedal, you are probably aware that it takes a ride or two to adjust to wearing them. And you might be thinking, "No one would be dumb enough to race in a new pair of clip-ins without having worn them before." No one except me, of course. And to exacerbate problems, a nor'easter had passed through the area the night before the race. I'm not talking about a late afternoon shower in Florida or the non-stop drizzle of Seattle, but heavy torrential sheets of the New England wet stuff. The rains left the race course a mud pit, literally.

I rode anyway, clip-ins and all, undeterred by the elements or the new equipment. The only thing I dreaded was the possibility I might come in last.

And I probably did. But I'll never know, as I didn't bother to look at the final standings (just in case). I almost threw up in the first 500 yards, and spend the majority of the race "on foot" rather than "on bike." But regardless of the dirty clothes and muddy face I had to show for it, I had a great time and was ready to try it again soon afterwards.

Your memory of a race will be the experience itself, not the place you finished. So don't worry about how well you do when you set out to conquer such challenges. Just *finishing* is an accomplishment.

## Don't Be Intimidated

After one of my many unsuccessful dating relationships during my 30s, I decided to pedal my way out of heartbreak. (By the way, I totally recommend this over tears and/or alcohol.) I got a Western Spirit catalog and picked the hardest mountain bike tour they offered—a majestic, week-long ride on the Colorado Trail. I naively thought my $350 Trek bike would be ideal for the trip and paid $150 to ship it across the country, perhaps because it's hard to realize how bad a Ford Fiesta really is until you drive a BMW.

Upon arriving at the airport with my amateur ride, I was immediately greeted by fellow participants on the tour, each standing next to their $2,000 and $3,000 bicycles. They looked at me in dismay and asked with a hint of ridicule, "You're not riding with the group from Telluride to Durango, are you?" I later found out that a few of these participants were pro racers, and the only other female on the trip was a former Nevada state champ. "Oh boy," I thought to myself. "What have I gotten myself into?"

On the first day of our trip, all the riders took off from Telluride at breakneck, race-day speed, and I was wondering how I'd ever be able to complete the trip without slowing everyone else down and really embarrassing myself.

And truthfully, I was the slowest rider in the group, and I probably did look dumb as I collected more cuts and bruises than the rest of the group put together. But I held my own, even when I had to pitch my own tent each night (a task almost as challenging as the ride itself). I ended up having a wonderful experience that made a lasting impression. For the years that followed, when a life catastrophe struck, I would always ask myself, "Remember that Colorado trip? If you can do that, you can do anything."

So don't be intimated, embarrassed or overwhelmed by an event or challenge. There's a reason why Nike's slogan is "Just do it" and not "Win at any cost."

# KICK IT UP A NOTCH

I have lots of endurance and very little speed. In fact, my 10K pace is not much faster than my marathon pace. And because I have never really been all that fast, I have a good excuse to continue running slowly. This philosophy serves me well when I'm training—if I run too hard, it won't be fun or I'll get injured and might have to stop doing it altogether.

The only problem with this philosophy is sticking to it on race day. I can't resist competing with faster runners so I nearly kill myself, all while my times get slower and slower. How could this be? I can't blame it solely on old age.

So, I'm trying out a new philosophy:

**You'll never run faster unless you start running faster.**

As I already mentioned, I started experimenting with speed workouts while trying to qualify for the 2009 Boston marathon, and admittedly, they were, and still are, as miserable as spending an entire day at work making cold calls. About the only good thing about these exhausting workouts is that the endorphin rush is more dramatic than after a long, slow run. So after my speed workouts, I feel like a million bucks. And there's more: though I'll never be a Marion Jones (even a Marion Jones before the steroids), my times are gradually improving.

Yours will, too, regardless of the sport. So pick up the pace. Even if you don't like the way it feels during, you'll definitely like the results after.

# DON'T FORGET TO STRETCH

How many times do you hit the gym or go for a walk and race home to shower and move on with your day? Do you play a tennis match with your friends and immediately congregate for the latest gossip, snack and glass of wine? That's certainly what we do in my tennis league.

Though I'm often guilty of not following my own advice, I do recommend deep, long stretches after every workout. And not the kind my husband does, when he bends down for a second or two and claims he stretched for a *long* time. Get into the stretch and hold it, maybe even for as long as 60 seconds, depending on the body part. Time goes by slowly when you are stretching, so watching the clock is helpful to ensure you are holding the stretch as long as you think you are.

Another thing to keep in mind is that it is better if you are warmed up when you stretch; otherwise, you might pull a cold muscle. If you don't have time to engage in a full-fledged workout to warm up, then walk while gently pumping your arms, or do a favorite exercise at low intensity for five to 10 minutes before stretching. And—don't bounce during a stretch. Whoever started that practice anyway?

What makes stretching such a good idea? I'll give you just a few of the many reasons.

**Stretching increases flexibility.** I've already mentioned that flexibility is one of the five components of fitness, but why? For one, increased flexibility can improve your daily performance, whether you are picking a pen off the floor or walking to the train station. Second, it can help reduce the risk of muscle, joint and tendon injuries. As you get older, your muscles shorten and tighten (while everything else in your body seems to be loosening up). As a result, you move more slowly, walk less straight and stiffen up more easily. This increases your chances for injury, unless you stretch those muscles, joints and tendons back out after working them.

**Stretching improves circulation.** Increasing the blood flow to your muscles helps supply them with the nutrients they need and helps remove the waste they collect from a strenuous workout. This means you can recover more quickly from workouts and heal injuries faster.

**Stretching can relieve stress.** By relaxing tense muscles, you help alleviate the tension that accumulates during a hectic day. Stretching is also a great way to give yourself a time out when you need one.

**Stretching improves the range of motion of your joints.** Balance and flexibility decrease with age, explaining, in part, why elderly men and women often fall and break a hip. Good range of motion keeps you moving and in better balance, thus making you less prone to falls and potential injuries. I don't know about you, but I don't need to wait until I'm 70 to do something to prevent falls, especially given my high klutz factor. So I'm stretching right now.

**Stretching can alleviate lower back pain.** Many of us are limited in our ability to move and exercise because of this common ailment. Often, low back problems are caused by muscle tightness in the quadriceps, hamstrings, hip flexors and low back muscles. Stretching these muscles can help eliminate the back pain, or at least lessen it.

If you don't know how to stretch properly, it's worth taking the time and trouble to find someone who does. That could be a certified trainer, an employee at the gym or your old track coach. And if you find yourself getting bored doing the same stretch routine on a daily basis, try Pilates or yoga. Yoga tones your muscles and increases flexibility, while Pilates improves your range of motion, flexibility, circulation, posture and abdominal strength.

You can stretch anytime, anyplace. If you take deep breaths while you're at it, you'll experience even greater benefits. So what are you waiting for? Reach down and touch those toes.

# HIRE A PERSONAL TRAINER

A few years ago, I hired training extraordinaire Karrie Wood to work with me for a few months. I knew I liked Karrie when I declared on our first day of working together, "Look, I have to tell you before we get started that I love sweets and my glass of wine at night. So I may not be your ideal client."

Her response was: "Good. If you didn't drink wine or eat sweets, I wouldn't want to work with you." Now that's my kind of trainer!

The other thing I learned from her right off the bat was that to attain the perfect movie star body, and specifically to have washboard abs, you must be prepared for a commitment as strenuous as a marathon. It takes a rigorous, no-excuses combination of diet, strength training and cardio to build muscles, keep the tendons flat and minimize subcutaneous fat. Who wants to go to that much trouble?

I started working on my abs as a means of strengthening my core and protecting my back, not just for the sake of appearance. After all, if your bottom is already starting to sag, what do a few stomach rolls matter? I have battled back problems for years, and having a child only exacerbated the issue. I am determined to continue mountain biking and skiing without letting an aching back stand in the way.

Karrie designed a workout plan, heavily based in Pilates, to strengthen this otherwise weak part of my body. Even though I no longer work with her on a regular basis, I still do many of the exercises she recommended.

A personal trainer can design a fitness routine tailored to your unique body, lifestyle and nagging pains. They can help you incorporate techniques that prevent problems which might arise down the road. They can keep you in shape and motivate you to stay healthy and toned. And they do all this in a structured, safe way. Another bonus? Sometimes a personal trainer might even save you a doctor bill or two. Karrie offered advice about my husband's injured calf and saved him a $150 doctor visit.

At the very least, a personal trainer (much like a business coach) will hold you accountable to the fitness goals you have set out to accomplish. And even the most disciplined among us often need that kind of accountability to stay on track.

So how do you find the trainer who's right for you? As with any health provider, word of mouth is probably the number one source. There are thousands of certifications, so it may be difficult to measure the credibility of one versus another. The National Academy of Sports Medicine is very reputable, so you might search for a trainer who is NASM certified. You can also visit www.acefitness.org to find ACE-certified trainers in your area.

Just remember, finding the right personal trainer is a lot like finding the right therapist. It's important that their approach and personality mesh well with yours. Some trainers motivate through encouragement and others by breaking people down. Make sure you find one who suits your style and helps you get results. It may take more than one attempt to get there.

Hiring a personal trainer is no small investment, but the payoff is tremendous and the benefits can last the rest of your life.

# MAKE EXERCISE SOCIAL

Have you ever taken a personality test, perhaps as part of a job interview or management training class? I have tried several over the years and always score high on the extroverted scale. I enjoy the companionship of others and social stimulation is important to me, so I use that as a motivator to exercise.

But even if you are an introvert, there are many merits to exercising with others, turning it into a social event and challenging your own progress against that of a friend.

Exercise has become a social outlet for me and completes my life in more than one respect. As a friend termed it, social exercising is a "two-for." Perfect example: I now run with some of the coolest people on the planet, a group labeled Team Dirty Martini. Regardless of how painful the run is, I enjoy conversing with my friends, sharing our thoughts on life, business and politics. Even mindless gossip makes a group run far more enjoyable than a solo outing. I could never survive all those 20-milers without Jodi's entertainment and moral support!

Another bonus? Team Dirty Martini makes sure I rise and shine at 7 a.m. on summer Saturdays, leaving the rest of my weekend free for fun and feeling good. Since I have started training with them, I run faster, too. When you are exercising and conversing with others, you naturally pick up the pace without feeling quite as much of the pain. And when you run faster, you start running faster (sound familiar?).

Other social outlet-meet-exercise experiences are road trips, like the week-long ski adventures I already mentioned. During those weeks, we enjoyed a lot of fresh power, attempted to ski the trees and did really bad Jonny Mosely impressions while jumping small bumps and lids. We laughed when Mae Charles met us for happy hour in her brand new ski pants, though she hadn't skied a lick all day. And when Cam got sick on the chair lift one morning after a big night out. Though I once took a tumble down a double black diamond chute-turned-cliff, from which I miraculously recovered unscathed, we all survived the trips happier and healthier. (Thanks for catching me, Ted!)

Aside from group runs and trips, do you enjoy yoga but find yourself losing interest when you do the same routines to the same tapes over and over again? Even if you are watching an instructor on television, repetition can lead to monotony. Not only that, but practicing solo may result in improper poses, which defeats the purpose of doing them in the first place. There's something about taking a live class and showing up in person that results in deeper, longer poses, better stretches, and a more peaceful *Savasana* (otherwise known as "corpse pose"). Especially when I compare that experience to the kind I have at home with children banging on the door and dogs licking my face or farting.

Like yoga classes, team sports can also be motivating and fun. Whether you play on a tennis, soccer or basketball team, the bottom line is that others are counting on you, so you've got to show up. It's that accountability thing again. And there's almost always some kind of social hour when the game or match is over, making all the effort even more worthwhile. Especially if you are new to a city, taking up a team sport can be an ideal way to meet people and make friends. And in the process, you will have burned a calorie or two.

So whether it's yoga, tennis or jogging, trying doing it with others. Competition, stimulation and encouragement can dramatically improve the experience and compel you to stick with it.

# WORK ON WHAT HURTS

I went to the doctor a while back to inquire about a hip injury and he made the comment, "I have to work so hard just to be able to work out." After religiously adhering to his recommended physical therapy program for months on end, I now understand what he meant.

If you are 40 or under, you can probably skip this chapter. For most of us, things don't really start breaking down until age 40, unless you have a torn meniscus or other chronic injury. So why bother worrying about what may lie ahead? In the meantime, do your stretches and bask in the youthful joys of quick recoveries and minimal body aches and pains.

For those of us over 40, gone are the days when we could do a little extra stretching and recover from an injury. When we could crash on our mountain bikes and be back in the game by the next day. Or wear a jog bra without needing a shirt to cover up our bellies. My friend Cam and I used to wear ours when hiking, taking pictures of ourselves like we had abs of steel. Though we used to laugh about our sub-par BGs ("butts and guts") while sporting this rather revealing outfit, I'd give anything for the BG I had when I was 30!

Now that I'm past 40, I've come to accept preventive measures as a part of my life. Looking back with envy never does much to help heal my aching back or throbbing hip! I know how much I want to keep exercising as I age gracefully, so I'm willing to put in the extra time to stretch, tone and massage those body parts that need a little extra attention.

Here's my advice on staying healthy and healed after 40:

**Stretch**. I need not repeat a chapter's worth of information here. Hopefully you're convinced of the benefits of stretching for injury prevention and healing.

**Start slowly**. I don't mean to keep picking on my husband, but he's such an easy target! He only knows two speeds, a complete halt or a full-on sprint, whether he's biking or running or skiing. If that sounds like you, maybe you got away with it in your twenties, but now it's time to develop a novel habit called warming up! Gradually increase your heart rate and give those muscles a little time to wake up and react. It's such a simple concept yet so few of us bother to do it. When you hop out on the ski slopes, don't go straight for the black diamond bumps. Not only will it not kill you to warm-up on some slow, easy blue runs first, it may even save your back and legs for rest of the afternoon or week.

**Isolate problem parts**. Mine just happens to be my back, thanks to a mild case of scoliosis and my little guy Luke. Strengthening your core, especially the abdominals, typically helps prevent and alleviate back pains and aches. Strengthening the muscles in the upper leg area helps to realign knee joints. By focusing on critical muscles, you might spare yourself plenty of unnecessary pain.

**Sooth the injury**. Some injuries require time off for healing. Others can be "put into remission" by physical therapy. That's what I did with my hip injury while training for the Chicago marathon. I spent more time doing physical therapy for my hip injury than I did running; and even though the injury didn't go away, I was able to minimize the pain long enough to endure the 26-mile distance comfortably enough (at least until I bonked). Though runners like me are generally half crazy, what matters most is doing what I love, so I'm willing to find ways to manage the pain while I do it.

**Try something different**. If your foot hurts from running, then find an alternative sport which doesn't require the same use of your foot, such as biking. Water exercise is ideal for people with joint injuries affected by bearing weight, but swimming might not be great for someone who just tore his rotator cuff playing golf or baseball. I'm sure you get the picture. Find activities that use different body parts and muscles to give the ailing ones a break.

**Go see the doctor**. I have had great luck with sports medicine professionals who predominantly treat athletes and really understand their common injuries. They seem to understand immediately what the problem is and how to fix it, even without x-rays. A physical therapist will work with you and recommend a number of strengthening and stretching exercises to help heal the pain and learn better body mechanics. It works, especially if you do what they tell you!

**Get lots of massages**. When all else fails, this medicine is the best you can take. Who doesn't enjoy a massage, after all? And isn't it a lot easier to spend money on something more pleasurable than a doctor visit? Sometimes muscles get ridiculously tight when you pound them a little too frequently, and continuing to stress and strengthen an already tight muscle may not help. Loosening the muscles through massage often eases the pain and improves your performance. Or so the massage therapist tells me. And I don't argue; massages have helped my hip injury even more than physical therapy.

And on that relaxing note, why don't you schedule an appointment? Your over-40 body will thank you.

# START PUMPING IRON

Building muscles is not just for guys and body builders. It's an important part of every fitness program, regardless of gender, how old you are or what shape you're in. If you are not including strength training with your cardio workouts, then you are missing out on a critical component of your overall health and fitness.

The benefits of adding muscle strengthening exercises to your workouts are profound. Among them are looking better, feeling better and speeding up your metabolism. And that's just the start.

**Look better.** After the age of 30, your muscles begin to decrease in size and strength. Your physical appearance and performance improve if you strengthen your muscles; and conversely, if you lose muscle mass, your appearance and performance decline. If you don't do anything to replace lean muscle mass, then fat will take its place.

**Control your weight.** If you like to eat as much as I do, you probably look for ways to consume the foods you like and burn calories more efficiently. If your muscles are more toned, it's much easier to control your weight. Why? Because your basal metabolic rate (BMR), or the energy used by your body at rest to maintain normal body functions, increases as your muscle mass increases. The more muscle mass you have, the more calories you burn, even when you're sleeping or sitting around. Likewise, with less muscle and more fat, your BMR will decrease. So lift weights, and lose weight.

**Help reduce the risk of injury.** If you build muscle, you help project your joints and make them less susceptible to injury. Strong muscles also help keep you balanced so you're less likely to fall. In addition, well-conditioned muscles help cushion the impact of weight-bearing activities like running and basketball.

**Develop strong bones.** Strength training can increase bone density and reduce the risk of osteoporosis.

**Sleep better.** Hey, this one was news to me until I was doing research for this book. I'll try anything that contributes to a good night's sleep.

**Manage chronic illnesses.** Strength training can reduce the signs and symptoms of chronic conditions such as obesity, arthritis, back pain and depression, as well as osteoporosis.

If you don't know how to do strength training correctly, ask a physical therapist, take a class at your local gym or hire a personal trainer. There are many misconceptions about how to lift and it's easy to hurt yourself through poor technique. A qualified instructor or trainer will help you devise a safe and effective program to work the muscles you want to strengthen.

There are number of different ways to integrate strength training into your day, some that require a gym and some that don't.

**Body-weight exercises.** The best part about body-weight exercises is that you can do them anywhere, including on the road while you are travelling or at home while watching TV. Using your own weight as resistance, you can do push-ups, pull-ups, abdominal crunches and leg squats, just to name a few.

**Machine-weight exercises.** I have never been to a gym that didn't have resistance machines, and you can even buy one for your home. I'll never forget how much fun we made of a certain family member when he purchased his own Bowflex system to build sleek and sexy muscles. But he got the last laugh when it worked.

Weight machines encourage good form, because they limit the range of motion to the safe zone of a specified exercise you are performing. In addition, they allow you to use more resistance. The disadvantage of machine weights is that they don't engage stabilizer muscles or develop core strength and conditioning as well as free weights.

**Free-weight exercises.** Free weights, like barbells and dumbbells, offer more flexibility and more options in terms of movement and muscle groups. Many free-weight exercises engage additional muscle groups beyond the primary one being targeted. Free weights also allow you to make subtle adjustments in your movement and positioning, potentially yielding better results. The downsides of free weights are an increased potential for improper form and limitations on the amount of weight you can use.

Your muscles adapt very quickly to stress, so by mixing up the kind of muscle conditioning exercises you do, you can make more progress and reduce the risk of hitting a training plateau. Hmmm... sound familiar?

Don't forget to warm up for about five to ten minutes before lifting weights, and give yourself time to recover, at least a full day between workouts on a particular muscle group. You may notice an increase in stamina in as few as two weeks, simply from lifting two to three times a week for just 30 minutes.

If you make strength training part of your fitness routine, you'll be amazed at what it can do for your physical and emotional well-being.

# GET A DOG

I realize that not everyone is a dog person. Admittedly, I am biased because I love dogs and think they add a lot of joy to a household, especially after they are potty trained and no longer eat your furniture. They can lower blood pressure and make you feel loved, even on those days when everyone and everything else gets you down. They love you with no strings attached, and forgive you instantly when you have wronged them.

About the only time dogs seem to get mad is when you put them in a kennel during vacation or business trips. My loving yellow lab, Shelby, used to let me know how she felt about the kennel by peeing in the car on the way home.

But there's another great thing about dogs that is rarely mentioned in books or movies. They are great at getting your lazy butt off the couch. I can't count the number of times I have gone for a run just to take my dog along and wear him or her out. After all, a tired puppy is much more pleasant to have around than the stir crazy one chewing your socks and hiding your shoes.

One of my fondest memories of Shelby traces back to my days in Boston in the mid-nineties. I raised money for the Dana-Farber Cancer Institute to "earn" a number for the Boston marathon. Each Thursday night, team members of the DFMC (Dana-Farber Marathon Challenge) would take the train, or "T," out to Newton and run the marathon course into the Back Bay, straight to the Eliot Lounge. I always dragged Shelby with me on these excursions. Not only did the bartender take dutiful care of her, but she was my trademark sidekick among the running group and other friends.

There's also an added satisfaction in seeing your dog happy to be outside. For a brief moment, while exercising, you can actually forget the pain you are enduring while watching your furry friend pounce around in the grass with a look of total bliss on her face.

Even if you don't run, just getting out the door for a walk around the block is good for both you and the dog, especially if you live in a place like Seattle and need extra motivation to fight the dreary weather. Would you get up from a good book, a good glass of wine or a good movie to go for a walk otherwise? Would you go to the park to see the sights if you didn't have a dog to motivate you toward a change of scenery?

Dogs cheer you up, make you laugh (usually, at least) and keep you moving. And even if they don't have an obsession with the air like Shelby did, they'll lick you right into a state of bliss.

# Live It Up!

Who doesn't know what I'm talking about
Who's never left home, who's never struck out
To find a dream and a life of their own
A place in the clouds, a foundation of stone

Many precede and many will follow
A young girl's dream no longer hollow
It takes the shape of a place out west
But what it holds for her, she hasn't yet guessed

She needs wide open spaces
Room to make her big mistakes
She needs new faces
She knows the high stakes

Dixie Chicks, "Wide Open Spaces"

# THE CYCLES OF LIFE

In my marketing business, I spend a lot of time talking about product life cycles with clients; but when I think about it, human lives also move in cyclical patterns.

## Phase 1: Conception to College

This is a period when life's learning curve is especially steep. As we grow and learn, our innocent, loving nature gets a bit toughened by the people and events that surround us. We go from leaning on our parents for everything to wanting them around for nothing. We go from time-outs to being grounded. We go from sitting in their laps to driving their cars.

I am not sure if you found junior high as excruciating as I did. At the time, I was growing taller but not filling out. I had just about the ugliest hair you could find on the planet. And as many crushes as I might have had on boys, I couldn't get one to look at me to save my life. In fact, I was in junior high during the disco era, and the one time I actually attended one of these events, not a single boy asked me to dance the entire evening. I went home in tears, and my mom tried to console me by saying, "Melinda, your day will come."

And my day did come in high school, when I gained more confidence and wisdom and as my figure began to develop. And continue to develop. Right on into college when I added enough weight for two people.

Those pre-college years are so incredibly influential. During this period, so many people form lifelong images of who they are and how they should look.

What we all probably failed to appreciate at the time was how lucky we were to keep weight off more easily, exercise without getting hurt and sport a wrinkle-free complexion. I can hardly believe I used to sit in the sun slathered in iodine-infused baby oil to better absorb the sun's rays! But I did so religiously in high school, so that my legs were as tanned as my friend Sandy's. Didn't I have my priorities straight at the age of 18?

## Phase 2: The Single Life

For me, this portion of the cycle spanned nearly two decades; for others, it may only span a few years. My pre-marriage phase was heavily influenced by the work-hard-play-hard mentality. I was employed by a series of companies, switching jobs more than was advantageous for a girl's career in those days, and spent way too much time with a U-Haul van attached to my car. My Phase 2 was also characterized by drinking beers and kissing frogs, without a fear in the world that anything really bad might happen to me.

Before marriage, and especially before kids, the world revolves around us, not necessarily because we are selfish, but more because we only have ourselves to nurture. Right? We're not obliged to pick up anyone else's clothes off the floor. We don't have to fix dinner for anyone but yours truly. There's no one else to leave the toothpaste open to dry out. There's no one to interfere with our workout schedules (we only have ourselves to blame for wimping out). More importantly, no one is depending on us for food, clothing and shelter.

You can get up at 6 a.m. and leave for work right away if you feel like getting off to a head start. Or work late without having to get anyone's permission. You can go out of town at a minute's notice, and even see a movie without having to move the earth and spend a fortune to find a babysitter.

On the other hand, you may often end up sitting through that movie alone, debating that twisted plot with yourself and the Internet's finest movie resources. More importantly, when you get home from the theater, there'll be no little angel fast asleep in bed, awaiting the goodnight kiss he actually doesn't remember getting. Whether it comes from our DNA or from watching too many Meg Ryan movies, most of us have a powerful urge for pairing up. Often accompanied by the desire to reproduce.

## Phase 3: Marriage and Kids

Not only does it take a lot longer to clean the house and cook dinner in this phase, but it costs a heck of a lot more at the grocery store. Your life is no longer your own, and time alone is a rare and precious commodity. The rewards are well worth the sacrifices, but it does take some major adjustments to your schedule. It takes quite a bit more planning (to do pretty much anything). There are no more "free" movies and very few relaxing dinners. If you work outside the home during the day, you try to play catch up at night with your kids. If your job is to stay at home with the kids, you might even feel like you're starting to lose your own identity.

For me, I have learned to live with bags of Tostitos and Oreos in the pantry, a monumental exercise in self-control. I often have to schedule my workouts in the wee hours before anyone else in the house is awake, despite the fact I could never get myself out of bed in the 40 years prior. And I NEVER stay up late anymore. The party queen days are long gone.

Even if you never marry or have children, life takes its twists and turns as you get older. Especially when the table turns and your parents become the ones who need special care instead of you.

## Phase 4: The Fashionably Late Years

Life's "brevity," as John Grogan so eerily and accurately describes in *Marley and Me*, is so apparent in this phase of one's life cycle. Making the comparison between the human life and that of a dog, he suggests:

> "One day you're swimming halfway out into the ocean convinced this is the day you will catch that seagull; the next you're barely able to bend down to drink out of your water bowl."

Likewise, one day you're running everywhere you go, eager to catch the next glimpse of whatever is around the corner. The next day, arthritis and knee problems have made it hard to walk around the block. One moment, your belly is a bottomless pit; then before you know it, you can't look at a plate of food without gaining weight.

One day you're griping and complaining when someone tells you to do stretches before you exercise, but then suddenly you can't even touch your toes without pulling a muscle. You can't stay awake past ten to save your life, so you go to bed early, then experience insomnia. Once desperate to conquer the professional world, all you want to do now is retire.

Despite the wrinkles, dry skin and lack of flexibility, you have a wealth of wisdom ready to pass along to the next generation—if only someone were willing to take you seriously.

Though we each experience unique cycles in life, our individual circumstances influence our daily routines at every age, affecting our livelihood, health and happiness. When we reach watershed moments it's helpful to step outside these circumstances, appreciate them and maybe even think about modifying some of them rather than trying to swim upstream against the current of aging.

Things that made you happy and healthy at 25 are probably not the same things which make your life complete at 45 or 55. As you recognize and accept your own transitions, you'll figure out a well-being formula that works for you. Just keep in mind that it may take a little bit longer and require ingenious creativity. And you may need some reading glasses to keep track of the details on paper.

# FIND YOUR OWN BALANCE

I was a late bloomer in many ways. I didn't develop breasts until I was nearly 16 years old. I went from wearing no bra to needing a C cup during a single summer between my ninth and tenth grade years of high school. It was actually quite embarrassing, especially when John Freeman announced in front of a huge group of students, "It looks like Melinda has eaten silicone over the summer."

I couldn't solidify my college major until I had to declare one in college, and didn't own a couch until I was 26. I attended graduate school later than most, thus earning the nickname "grand mom" from my classmates. When I was 34 and had excelled fairly quickly at my Fortune 500 employer, the VP of marketing had to tell me to dress more professionally (that is, not to wear overalls to the office). I got married at age 39 and had my first and only child two weeks shy of my 40th birthday. And I'm still trying to figure out what I want to be when I grow up.

"What is your passion in life?" has been a common theme throughout my life. I've taken numerous personality tests, many career tests, read personal growth books and watched way too many *Oprah* episodes. I stand green with envy over the stories of men and women who somehow manage to find their passion, pursue it and make money along the way by doing what they love to do.

Since I was single for so long, and since I have always been a career-minded individual, it's not surprising that my job status and level of professional fulfillment greatly influence my happiness. I am sure there are many of you out there who feel similarly. But I am starting to learn, as I get older and wiser, that it takes more than a successful career to live a satisfying life.

Maria Shriver's *Just Who Will You Be?* wonderfully describes the exploration of personal identity. After moving to California for her husband's political ambitions and being asked to leave her job as a newswoman at NBC, she found herself wondering what she wanted to be when she grew up. After much soul searching, she finally realized she had been asking herself the wrong question. Rather than "what" she wanted to be, a question she had always answered with "my résumé," she should have been asking "who" she wanted to be.

To steal a line from the movie *Jerry Maguire*, what "completes" me now is different than what completed me 10 or 20 years ago. My lifestyle was different, the stakes were different, my skin far smoother and my figure more perky than it is now. Marriage and a child have taught me a lot about selfless love and gratification, and many other events through my life have shaped the person I have become as well.

A bad economy is a really good thing for a few reasons. If business is bad and finances are less secure, it forces you to look for and appreciate what really gives you comfort and meaning in life. If you're having a bad day, what is the one thing that makes you feel better? Is it a workout, a kiss from your spouse, and a hug from your child or ten minutes of meditation? Is it a good book, an unforgettable movie or a glass of wine with some friends?

No one can tell you where you get your comfort, or where you get your point of balance, fulfillment and security. It's a different formula for everyone. But it's important, I think, to try to figure out that formula. If you lost your job or your home, what couldn't you live without? What or who would make you happy? Take note of these precious gems and remember to be grateful for them, even when things are going smoothly.

For me, my family and my health are who and what matter most to me. No matter how bad my day has been, it can be temporarily erased by a hug from my son and the sound of his laughter. Though it's easy to take a relationship for granted, I am blessed to have the security and comfort of a loving husband who truly cares about me and my happiness. And I'm especially thankful that I am able to exercise. A little run, walk or bike ride does wonders to cure the blues, improve my spirits and restore my confidence.

This is my life's seesaw, the balance between professional and personal endeavors. If I place too much emphasis on career or money or other materialistic things, the seesaw tilts too far to one side. What keeps your seesaw from teetering dramatically up or down?

# *AND KEEP WORK IN PERSPECTIVE*

My husband and I recently hosted a dinner party for three other couples. It was an enjoyable evening filled with good food, even better wine and lots of laughter. Then, right after the main course, suddenly everyone whipped out their iPhones in unison.

Five people of the crowd owned an iPhone, and each of them was eager to share top-ranking apps, the fart game, how many calories they'd consumed and burned that day, and on and on. You know times are changing when you can't make it through a dinner without breaking out a telecommunications device.

I spent three years consulting with a Smartphone manufacturer, helping them grow their market share from virtually no distribution in the US to one which surpassed Palm. I wrote endless copy about how Smartphones can change a person's life: Stay in the know when you're on the go. Stay ahead of the game. Stay on top of business and personal matters. And my personal favorite: Now you can work 24/7. Ironically, for me, the question is who the heck really wants to work 24 hours a day, 7 days a week, either with or without a Smartphone?

I personally dislike the "crackberry" culture and the need to check e-mail, text messages and Facebook *all the time*. After all, what's the harm in a little face-to-face communication for a change? Though technology is often quite empowering and enabling (buzz words used way too often), there are times when I really want to return to the good old days. Days when we got home and played with our children instead of technology and its many gadgets.

One of my first bosses after grad school was a talented Harvard Business School alumnus. She was good at her job, very efficient and confident in her abilities. Early in my tenure working for her, she said to me very emphatically, "I work from 8 to 5. If I can't get my work completed in that timeframe, there is something wrong with the job, not with me."

I was surprised to see that this attitude didn't hold her back from accelerated career success and wondered why more people didn't adopt her approach. I know I did (for the most part, anyway), and found that her mantra goes a long way toward creating an enjoyable and balanced life.

During the dot-com era, my balance teetered out of control. When the CEO, my boss at the time, called a meeting at 8 p.m., I couldn't exactly tell him something was wrong with the job, not me, unless I was prepared to quit. These were days when I was stressed out a lot, had circles under my eyes and wasn't in the best of shape physically. More importantly, my dog Shelby was very lonely and spent needless hours waiting at home alone for her mom.

People worked around the clock to get everything done faster, regardless of how important (or not!) the work really was. The "quick cash, retire young" mentality grew old, especially as stock prices shrank and work hours continued to expand. During this time, I left corporate America and started my own company. Though getting my business off the ground required time and dedication, at least I could control my work hours, get some quality sleep and take my dog to work.

Though our professions are central to our lives and standard of living, there's more to life than work. I believe that careers are much more meaningful when we keep them in perspective. Even at my pinnacle of corporate success, I was single and had no one with whom to share my achievements (or at least someone who *really* cared besides my mom). As a small business owner, I have far fewer trophies to bring home from the office at night, but I have friends and family to share my ups and downs. In addition, the work I carry out for clients each day is far more fulfilling. This, for me, makes for a far richer life.

As social networks bring new possibilities to the Internet, and as Smartphones get smarter and more fun, it can be challenging to draw the line between our work and personal lives. For me, a love for children and the outdoors provides a great incentive to break for recess. We all need creative outlets, significant others, hobbies and interests outside the parameters of whatever we do for a living.

Even when I was single and theoretically could have worked around the clock if I had wanted, I still found my old boss's 8–5 rule a good one to follow. Now, with a small child, I *have* to be home by 5:00 because of my nanny's schedule. I can always take an e-mail time-out after he's asleep, and it brings me great peace to honor the precious time I get to spend at home by leaving the office and all its worries at 5:00.

You can be dedicated to your job and good at what you do and still have time left over to pursue interests, cook a good meal or take a relaxing walk. So turn off that iPhone and leave the laptop closed when you get home from work. Get a good night's sleep for a change. And in the morning when you wake up feeling refreshed, you'll wonder why you ever thought that 10 P.M. e-mail was so urgent.

# MORE IS NOT ALWAYS BETTER

Have you ever caught yourself thinking the grass is greener on the other side? Do you ever think life would be easier if you lived in a different house, earned more money, dated a nicer man or had a different job? If so, join the club.

It's embarrassing to admit how many times I changed jobs thinking the *next* one would be the perfect one. I thought I'd find my Mr. Right in Virginia. Then Boston, then Seattle. Now that I've found him, I've moved on to dreams of a 48" Viking stove and 61" soaking tub (complete with overhanging chandelier).

How do overblown expectations become so integral to our very being, especially considering that high expectations are often inversely related to desirable outcomes? Some of my biggest disappointments occurred when reality failed to live up to my fantasies. When you're constantly looking to find a better job, meet a nicer guy or have a nicer home, you tend not to appreciate the perfectly fine job, guy or house you currently have. Where is the happiness in that?

There are many great writers and philosophers who would offer this advice in a much more eloquent way, but my motto is:

**Go with the flow, and let go!**

If you have children, you can learn to appreciate how events rarely proceed according to plan, especially if you are on vacation or planning a nice dinner out. Even a dog can teach you how not to get too attached to the idea that your furniture and shoes will always look nice if you take good care of them. When things go awry at work, try to appreciate the comedy of errors instead of getting worked up to the point of being completely ineffective. After all, if mishaps never occurred, how would we learn to do things differently or better?

By focusing less on what you wish for, and placing more emphasis on accepting "what is," you'll experience far fewer disappointment and let-downs. The sooner you can let go of an imaginary life where everything is perfect, the more you'll start enjoying the life you have right now.

# SLOW DOWN

We all inherit a selective combination of genes from our parents. The ones I got from my dad are the equivalent of "Energizer bunny" genes. Even at the age of 72, he rarely stops working on something. And me? I was a squirm worm at the age of six, and little has changed since those early days. I find it challenging to sit still and relax; I can always find something to do. As a result, "bored" is a rare word in my vocabulary.

I have created countless New Year's resolution lists which included "slow down," without success. I start out doing pretty well during the month of January, but by February I am racing around again. Somehow there are always excuses to hurry up, cram as much activity as possible into a given time period and then go, go, go.

Before I had a family, it was a professional commitment, sporting event or social engagement that kept me running; and since having a child (and a puppy), there's scarcely a moment when something doesn't need to be picked up, put up or cleaned up. Who has time to rest?

I've bought books about meditation and about how to live in the moment and taken numerous yoga classes in hopes of settling down and relaxing. But despite considerable effort, this is something I still struggle with and probably always will. And from what I see around me, I don't think I'm alone in this quandary.

Though having a child has added a lot to my list of things to do and remember, it's also the thing that most makes me want to slow down and take notice of extraordinary moments amidst ordinary circumstances. Even without kids, we all have many opportunities to stop and smell the roses, help a friend in need, write a note to someone who's lonesome or bask in the sun on a brisk autumn day.

The challenge is learning to slow down, with discipline and awareness, much like the skills required to eat well and exercise regularly.

**You won't learn to slow down until you slow down.**

If your heart is racing over a work deadline or you're getting exhausted doing the laundry, fixing dinner and picking up toys, all at the same time, the best medicine is to stop and take a deep breath.

Sometimes, one breath will do the trick and at other times you may need four or five. Even if you aren't breathing in the precise methodology taught in magazines or meditation classes, a simple pause to relax and reflect has an immediate calming effect.

I'm doing my best to take a dose of my own medicine and learn how to meditate. It's not easy. I find the practice daunting and feel rather embarrassed that I'm so bad at it, but it helps to cut myself some slack. I used to think I'd failed miserably at meditation if my mind wasn't completely at rest. Now I've given up on such a notion. Every time I shut my eyes, my mind races to the groceries I need to buy or things I forgot to do at work. I'm learning to accept my busy mind and calm it down as best I can. At least if I sit still and close my eyes, I am relaxing and slowing down.

I heard excellent advice about meditating on *Oprah*. One of her guests recommended starting with one minute of meditation each day during the first month of new practice, extending it to two minutes in the second month, three in the third, and so on. I like this advice because it sounds more attainable and habit-forming. As the months proceed and the meditation periods lengthen—and the pressure to be perfect eases up—meditation becomes an integral part of your day.

So rather than slowing down for resolution's sake, try making it a life-long habit. Sit down, slow down and enjoy the moments life has to offer. After all, even the Energizer bunny's batteries wear out sooner or later.

# APPRECIATE YOUR SPOUSE

I spent my twenties and thirties with grandiose visions of marriage as a never-ending blissful adventure with your soul mate. Marriage was to be a bright beacon amidst a fog of despair, a pinnacle on the mountain climb of life.

That was before the dirty clothes got thrown on the floor and the arguments over what to watch on TV, whose turn it is to do the dishes and which movie to go see.

In "The Scientist," Coldplay suggests, "Nobody said it was easy." Will Smith, in a recent interview, said, "Marriage is the hardest job you'll ever have." And I agree with both assessments. Marriage is work. It's trial and error. It's getting to know another person, how to support him, communicate with him and understand his moods. And vice versa. It's give and take. Compromise. Throwing in the towel and admitting you might be wrong every now and then.

Marriage has accentuated my own faults, shortcomings and imperfections. It has highlighted annoying behavior I never really thought about until someone else had to live with it day in and day out. And, unlike most parents, a spouse usually won't hesitate to tell you just how annoying this behavior truly is.

It definitely takes two to tango, and two to tangle.

Despite the challenges, however, marriage is comforting and rewarding. It's a rallying force against the world. It gives you a sense of belonging. It has alleviated the loneliness I once believed was an inevitable part of life years ago. And it means I no longer have to race to the video store on Friday nights to beat the crowds for bestselling movies.

My husband believes in who I am (though sometimes he shows it in weird ways), supports my decisions (though he may frequently disagree with them) and is my biggest cheerleader (despite the fact he won't go near a marathon course anymore). I know I have a friend no matter what happens.

It can be easy to forget this. Amid the hectic days of our lives, it's easy for spouses to neglect marriage and each other. We take so much time to work on that report at work, practice that sales pitch or prepare for that interview. We certainly don't forget to feed and clothe our children. But carving out the time to nurture our marriages usually falls to the bottom of the list, if it's even on the list.

In my own case, I have to check in regularly and ask myself, if I can lead team meetings once a week at work, why can't I just as easily schedule a date night once a week? Or even lunch together? I can't even remember the last time I went on a trip with my husband—without our child or parents accompanying us. When marriage reaches the doldrums, it's up to each of us to take responsibility for spicing things up again.

One challenge in our marriage is the scarcity of activities that first drew us together. When we first met, we were always planning a bike ride, going for a run and heading to the mountains for a ski or hike. Then we got pregnant just one month into our marriage. Becoming parents turned our outdoor lifestyle upside down. We suddenly found ourselves stuck *inside* the house.

We haven't necessarily figured out the perfect formula for working spontaneity and four-hour bike rides back into our routine. After all, a person can only afford so many sitters. And there are only so many play dates that happen to fall on Saturday mornings just as the sun is rising over the hills.

But we're learning. And working on it. And figuring out how to nurture our relationship while simultaneously raising a chatty child and training frisky dogs. I suppose this is what marriage is all about.

No matter what, I'm thankful for my spouse and the stability he brings to my life. And I'm learning to invest time and effort into this relationship, as I have with my career for so many years, giving it the attention it needs and deserves.

And what about you? Is your spouse a job, a hobby or an afterthought?

# ENJOY YOUR CHILDREN

My next book may be titled, *How to Be Happily Imperfect Parents*. At a time when TV shows, blogs and books are teaching us more and more about how we are supposed to teach, feed, discipline and love our children, how is it possible to live up to the world's expectations?

I'm sure our preschool teachers think my husband and I are the most forgetful parents on earth. No matter how many notes and reminders they send, we invariably forget Sound Share day and lose track of scheduled events (and the food items we were supposed to bring to those events).

And even though we have done extensive research on where to send our son for kindergarten—we spent as much time researching kindergartens as I did colleges—our efforts seemed to pale in comparison to those of other parents we know.

My little guy is often wearing pants that are two inches too short. I have never ironed an article of clothing for him. I buy him toys when I take him to Target just so he'll behave long enough for me to get what I went in for. I'm embarrassed to admit how many bags of chips and fruit rollups I have purchased at the grocery store when I take him. I even forced French fries down him years ago when he simply wouldn't eat anything (after swearing that no child of mine would ever be allowed to eat fried food). He drinks water from the dogs' bowls and eats their food when I'm not looking (and probably their treats, too).

Despite the big "S" (for sucker) I often wear on my forehead, I do at least limit his TV and computer time. I only give him sweets if he finishes his meals first, primarily because sugar makes him somewhat psychotic on an empty stomach. I always try to provide a balanced meal at dinner and have played enough games of Chutes and Ladders for eight kids. I play hide-n-seek before school and place Easter eggs around the house for him to find, even in the middle of summer. I sing to him (to which he now responds, "Mom, please stop") and dance with him (since his dad won't dance with me). I tickle his back and make up silly stories each night when I put him to bed. And I remember to bathe him (his father, on the other hand…).

I know I could never love anything or anyone more than I love my child. And I'd sacrifice anything in the world for him. There has never been a single thing in my life which has brought me more joy than he. The look on his precious face when he's asleep is one I always cherish. When he gets up in the morning and wants to sit in my lap, it's the best five minutes of my day. When he leaps into my arms when I get home from work, all the troubles of the world melt away. His "I love you's" mean more than life itself to me. And if I could capture his laughter in a jar, I would save it until eternity.

Children bring warmth, love and balance to life like nothing else in the world. Though I was only able to have one child due to my late-in-life start, others are unable to have kids at all. However, we can still appreciate and learn from the innocence, kindness and loving spirit of children. They remind us what it used to be like to be appreciative of almost anything, blissfully happy for no reason and entertained by so little. Who else could spend hours in the back yard mixing dirt with water with such intensity and interest (especially when there's a worm in the mix)?

So try to get a kid fix any way you can. And appreciate your own children while they're young. They'll be all grown up before you know it.

# LEARN A FEW THINGS FROM MOM

I liked the movie *Spanglish*, despite its not-so-hot reviews. After much turmoil, Flor (played by Paz Vega) refuses to allow her daughter Cristina (Shelbie Bruce) to attend the same private school as the children of the family she works for. She asks her daughter at the movie's end, "Is what you want for yourself to become something very different than me?" Though none of us wants to be a carbon copy of our mother or father, do we ever really become someone completely different?

Like the character in the movie, I grew up in a single-parent household. My parents divorced when I was young, so I had a strong estrogen influence in my upbringing. This generally meant a lot of running around in skimpy clothes, far too many emotional outbursts and plenty of cabinets, appliances and toys that broke and rarely got fixed. Go figure: after marriage, I'm in a house of all boys.

Over the years, I have learned to appreciate the accomplishments—and imperfections—of my mom in raising me. Moms have their own special way of:

- Making you feel loved.
- Lending a listening ear (even if she is tired of hearing about it).
- Offering a shoulder to cry on, even when the problem is inconsequential and unimportant.
- Providing advice on issues ranging from work to marriage to decorating houses.
- Giving your children way too much candy.
- Always remembering holidays, even the Hallmark ones you'd like to forget.

My mom, in particular, taught me values and lessons which will always stay with me, such as:

- Count your blessings.
- It's always darkest before the dawn.
- Always look on the bright side.
- Your day will come.
- Always trust that God is looking out for you.

Though I'm still somewhat bitter that she didn't tell me how bad my hair looked at many stages in my life, I still appreciate the many, many things she did well. She never harassed me when I did something wrong or fell short of her expectations because she knew I was harder on myself than anyone else could ever be. She let me make up my mind for myself, because she respected how independent I was. She stood back and watched me make mistakes, because she knew it was the only way I'd learn. And then there's the one that must have been hardest: she didn't express her opinion when I was dating someone she thought I shouldn't, giving me the chance to figure it out for myself (and I did, *eventually*).

Mothers have a nice way of convincing us of our superior intellect, above-average writing skills, exceptional athletic ability, good looks and amazing personality. Even though we know it's not true all the time (just most of the time), the encouragement was and is always welcome. After all, without her encouragement, we may not have become who we are today.

Now that I'm a parent, I realize how hard it is to do everything right. I can be much more forgiving and understanding about the way my mother raised me. She made mistakes, just like I will and already have. She didn't always know best, but she loved me without question, without criticism and without constraint. She worked hard and demonstrated courage.

A mother's influence is lasting and her support is often incomprehensible. And though I will never be as thoughtful and generous as my mom, I admire the positive impacts she has on others each day.

What life lessons can you thank your mother for?

# VALUE YOUR FRIENDS

I moved away from home when I was 18 to attend college. I left the South at age 30 and have never returned, except for family visits or vacations. Friends became family to me as I moved farther and farther away from home and spent more and more years trying to find someone who would marry me. Without my friends, I'm not sure how I would have survived.

Anyone who has moved far from home can attest to the important role friends play in our lives. And even those with parents and childhood friends a few blocks down road still need friends for comfort, support, laughter and mischief. Friends are irreplaceable for so many reasons.

Before marriage, they will:

- Let you cry on their shoulders after a break-up.
- Keep you company so you don't have to be alone on weekend nights.
- Eat the food you cook and almost always tell you how good it is (but then, nobody turns down a free home-cooked meal).
- Challenge you to an extra beer on a night out.
- Possibly even dance on the tabletops with you when you've had one too many.
- Better yet, take your keys away from you so you can't drive home.
- Tell you when you're dating someone who's not good enough (which is a good thing since you wouldn't listen if your parents told you).
- Take care of your dog when you go out of town, sometimes (though I don't hold it against my friends who once declined to take care of Shelby; really, I don't...)

- Talk you into athletic events you would have never tried otherwise (right, Bill?).
- Keep you company while you're exercising to alleviate the pain and tedium.
- Tell you if a new hair cut is really bad.
- Or if an outfit you're wearing is too tight, ugly or frumpy.
- Take vacations with you, which is really nice if you're not dating anyone.
- Get in all kinds of trouble with you.
- Come visit you when you live in fun cities, and almost miss their flights on the way home.
- Show up early when you have parties, reassuring you that others will arrive eventually.
- Even help you move if you buy them lots of beer.

After marriage, they will:

- Be a source of sanity when you need a break from your spouse and kids.
- Listen to your rants and help you realize that everyone goes through the same issues in life.
- Make you feel better when you realize you're not the only one who can't remember anything.
- Give you parenting advice when you wonder how you could ever have been put in charge of a little one.

Young or old, married or single, your friends will still talk you into exercising and even accompany you, eat your food and praise it, bring you up when you're down and celebrate with you when times are good.

Friends have an amazing way of letting you know you're special. They'll remind you of the often-forgotten gifts you have to offer the world. Ask them sometime to write down or even tell you how you have influenced their lives; their remarks might surprise you. I did this once with a small handful of close friends, and I still keep and cherish the words they wrote (especially Allen's, whose comments still make me cry).

A dose of friendship goes a long way in making life interesting, zany and sane, all at the same time. Without friends, life gets out of whack and off balance. Are you carving enough time out of the day for yours?

# GET STIMULATED

All of us manage to tax our brains at work. Whether you are selling stocks, balancing financial statements, writing advertising copy or selling medical equipment, you manage to use your noggin on a daily basis. And though some of you may be stuck in a rut in your current career and therefore argue my point, every job involves at least some aspects that are either intellectually stimulating or personally motivating.

But, regardless of how stimulated you are on the job, it's advantageous to exercise your intelligence and creativity outside of work hours, too. How you accomplish this is really up to you.

For some, it is as simple as reading a book; for others, it may require taking a course at a local community college. Others may need to pull out a blank canvass and paint until the wee hours of the morning. Regardless of what it takes, using your brain outside of the four walls of your office or cubicle is surprisingly restorative.

When I lived in bigger cities, the opportunities were limitless. From community colleges to university extension courses to museums and symphonies, I never had to worry about keeping my mind busy. In smaller towns you may have to look harder, but there will almost always be events to attend and courses to take. And if you can't find a class you like, you can figure out how to teach it yourself.

When I taught marketing at Seattle University on an adjunct basis, I learned far more from my students than they learned from me. And teaching doesn't have to mean working with college kids, either. My husband has regularly taught segments at our child's preschool and even the teachers belly up to hear what he has to say. He considers these opportunities to share and learn with children to be the brightest moments of his week.

And classes aren't the only opportunity to learn. There are so many ways to stimulate your mind. Several of my family members are talented at sewing and crafts. Unfortunately, I wasn't blessed with this skill, but I often try anyway. It may simply be another decade before I prepare home-made vinegars and oils for Christmas presents again.

My mother-in-law is gifted at renovating and decorating homes; my father at fixing just about anything in the house or yard that might be broken. I have numerous friends who knit, and others who are talented at photography. One of my all-time favorite employees, Jason, is launching a new business to market his photography, a creative interest he pursues on the side.

I am always amazed by the talents of others and the gifts they are able to offer the world by taking advantage of a little spare time, creativity and intellectual capacity.

If you seek, you shall find an array of ways to stimulate your mind. Not only will you enjoy the diversion, you'll also become a more well-rounded person in the process.

# ENTERTAIN YOURSELF

The line between stimulation and entertainment is blurry, but we all need opportunities to tune out and escape. A good book offers hours of pleasure *and* stimulation. I suppose a chick lit selection might fall more in the entertainment class, while a book about branding might be more intellectually fulfilling (in theory at least). Either way, it's easy to get lost in a good book.

Movies offer another great opportunity for escape. If you are down in the dumps or just need to get your mind off work at the end of the day, a movie captures the imagination and takes you to a place outside your immediate reality. Movies inspire, influence opinions, educate you on issues and even let you enjoy the competitive spirit of Oscar season. And if you and your spouse can't settle on a selection that pleases both your tastes, you can always go alone or meet a friend. Some of my fondest memories of Boston are of the many escapades with Marcia to see indie flicks.

Growing up in a region of the country where spectator sports abound, I can't help but get revved up by a good college basketball or football game. Those who live in an area of the country with a good professional franchise team can no doubt relate on a similar level. Going to school in Chapel Hill definitely contributed to my love for sports. Once when my brother-in-law was in town visiting, my friends and I had gathered to watch a Tar Heel basketball game. Upon observing our intensity, he exclaimed, "I have never in my life seen girls who know so much about basketball!"

Games are entertaining in more ways than one. I've met some wonderful people in Boise through the Duke/UNC basketball rivalry. In fact, my son's best friend is the daughter of "Dukies," a couple we originally met after she bit his ear (the rivalry started early).

Spectator sports have a nice way of diverting your thoughts from worries about work, finances or what you're going to fix for dinner.

However, watching sports shouldn't replace participating in them, so be careful about how much television time you are accumulating.

Speaking of games, I have played endless rounds of Candy Land with my five-year-old. Even though what I remember as being one of the greatest games on earth can now put me into a coma, I can still appreciate the simple pleasures of a board game, pair of dice or deck of cards. And as much as computer games scare me at times, I have seen with my own eyes how a Wii or *Guitar Hero* can entertain people for hours. Games can educate, harness some healthy competition and relieve stress.

Before my husband and I got married, we signed up for a wealth training seminar hosted by T. Harv Eker. Though some of the antics of the weekend were a bit much for me at times, especially the one where you had to get a little too excited about finding a penny on the ground, I found one aspect of the training particularly valuable. Eker advocated an approach to saving money which included time and funds set aside for entertainment. I have always believed that making time for fun is necessary to enhance a person's happiness, but the idea of setting aside money from each paycheck for entertainment, much like allocating cash for food, rent and savings, was new to me. We've been practicing it ever since.

# EXPLORE THE WORLD

Travelling is certainly one of my passions in life. Seeing and learning about other places, cultures and people is an experience like no other. Though travel may cause you to wish for a way of life you may never have, it can also help you appreciate the many blessings that come your way on a daily basis.

Whether it's a vacation, a honeymoon or time off between jobs, I highly recommend you get out there and explore the world. Travelling to a small town, big city or foreign country has a wonderful way of broadening your horizons. Taking a break and getting away can relax your mind, charge your batteries and brighten your outlook on life (except, perhaps, for those first few days of re-entering reality).

And don't let finances stop you—traveling doesn't have to mean spending a fortune. What about seeing the sites that are close to home, wherever you live?

Some of my favorite trips have been visits to small towns on the way to or from a mountain bike ride. Having a beer at a local pub provides a wonderful opportunity to get a snapshot of someone else's rituals and priorities. Even a place that's close in geographic proximity may be miles away from the life you lead.

My in-laws have learned so much about the country thanks to the endless miles they have put on their car, traversing the country and stopping in little towns along the way. They've used their travels as a great way to grow closer through new and different experiences together.

Bike rides are another great way to explore the landscape and really get to know it. As a bonus, you'll save money on gas and even on hotels if you camp along the way. A word about camping, though—it's not for everyone. While it's true that you'll never see the sky or smell the fresh air from a hotel room the way you can from a tent in the woods, the downside is that, in a tent, you will also have to smell your dirty selves.

My husband and I decided to camp during our honeymoon to extend our budget and our vacation. It wasn't exactly romantic. I spent more time dreaming about a hot shower than I did appreciating the extra three days we spent in Hawaii. Based on my experience, I'd suggest thinking through the pros and cons before committing to camping as a vacation option!

No matter where you lay your head at night, exploration is a sensation.

# GET IN TOUCH WITH YOUR SPIRITUAL SIDE

If you have ever been to the South, you'll notice there are churches on almost every corner of every block. Big churches, small churches. Beautiful churches and ugly ones. And you better believe, come Sunday, those pews will not be vacant. Going to church isn't optional in the South; you're expected to be there.

For my part, I have always thought, and still do, that going to church is a personal choice. You go because you want to hear a good sermon. You attend because you want to support the youth group. Or maybe because you want to meet other individuals who share common beliefs. Church was an important part of my youth, and it continues to start my week with an inspiring and optimistic lift (when I actually get myself and my family motivated to attend). I feel blessed to have a wonderful preacher six blocks from my house whom my friends have termed "Bill Clinton" because of his amazing ability to captivate an audience.

I believe in God and am a Christian. I truly believe there's Someone watching out for me. Someone taking care of me. Someone keeping me safe. And Someone who has my best interests at heart. My faith is nothing I can prove, but isn't that the point?

I've never been one to wear my religious heart on my sleeve, however. Outside of church I try to demonstrate my beliefs through actions and behavior, not by preaching to other people about God. I realize that many Christians will disagree with my hands-off approach. After all, how can you help others if you aren't willing to share your feelings on how the world was created, a higher purpose in life or the fleeting fulfillment of material rewards?

But I feel strongly that a person's religion or personal belief system is unique to that person. When I think about the people I've met in my life, the ones I view as the kindest, most giving or most forgiving aren't necessarily the ones who go to church the most. Or the ones who profess to be the most religious.

This is where I think spirituality comes into play. Being spiritual can be more meaningful than being religious. It might offer more solace than going to church. Being spiritual might provide a higher purpose to your life, even if God—or another deity—works slowly to illuminate your path to purpose.

Often, when I'm flying in an airplane, high above the clouds, I think about the many, many people below and how, from a great distance, they start looking like ants in a colony. When I'm on the ground, my own life is so significant; it's the center of the universe. But when I am high above the landscape, it's easier to view my life as being one small part within the context of many others.

Finding your spiritual side has many benefits for the heart, the soul and the body. It can be a tie that binds a relationship. And a comfort to parents in knowing a higher power is watching over their children. It helps us believe that everything happens for a reason and to accept things we don't understand. It's an explanation for why we have been blessed with treasures we may not feel we deserve. It helps comfort us in times of need. A spiritual perspective can unravel the knots in your stomach and even cleanse your thoughts of worries, hatred and grudges.

Removing such negative influences, in my opinion, improves your overall health and well-being. After all, if someone is spending so much time pent up in frustration, vindication and hatefulness, how could they possibly be filled with happiness, good health and good will for others or themselves?

For me, I feel the presence of a Higher Power whenever I cross the finish line of a marathon. Now, I realize that fatigue influences my ability to think clearly, but the accomplishment of completing a long distance run fills me with indescribable sentiments. This is why I feel blessed to be able to do these crazy races.

For months on end, I carry out those dreaded speed workouts and log 20-mile runs in snow and wind, wondering why I am putting my body through such torture. During the race itself, I play mind games for hours on end to fight the pain. If I hit the wall somewhere late in the race, I might even lose all coherence for awhile. But like I just experienced in Boston as I reached the Back Bay and turned onto Boylston Avenue with the finish line in view, the crowds and cheering suddenly seem larger than life. A mix of inspiration, appreciation and accomplishment wash over my body like the wind beating against it. And that's when I know I'm not alone, ever.

# *Afterword*

**Reasons to Ignore Everything You've Just Read:**

I'm too busy.

I'm not a good enough athlete.

I'm just going to wait until a doctor tells you to change.

I'm already skinny enough.

I want a faster, easier way to get healthy.

I am already happy enough.

**Reasons to Try at Least One or Two of My Ideas:**

**I am too busy.** We always manage to make time to do what we really want to do, when it comes down to it. The only person who can fit healthy habits into your day is you. You are welcome to all of my suggestions, but what's more important is that you find you own secret sauce.

**I am not a good enough athlete.** You'll always find someone who is a better athlete, a better cook, a better writer or a better salesperson than you'll ever be. But who cares? You're probably better than many others at a lot of things. All that really matters is that you engage in activities that make you feel good.

**I am just going to wait until a doctor tells me to change.** A doctor can't make you miraculously healthy any more than a CEO can tap you on the shoulder and make you instantly wealthy. Sure, a doctor can prescribe pills or perform surgery, but wouldn't it be safer, cheaper, and more rewarding to take charge of your own well-being and maybe even prevent health problems altogether? There will always be health issues you can't control, but why not proactively improve the way you feel without waiting for a doctor's orders?

**I am already skinny enough.** Being skinny is not the end goal of well-being. In fact, a slimmer, more toned figure should be a by-product of all the other healthy habits you have embraced. So forget all this nonsense about how being skinny is all that counts and switch your focus to being healthy. And happy.

**I want a faster, easier way to get healthy.** Your own well-being can't be bought or packaged. It's not a drive-through process or quick fix. Living well is a long-term commitment, a step-by-step establishment of little habits that add up to a big life. Like anything in life worth having, it takes time and attention and a willingness to laugh at yourself sometimes.

**I am already happy enough.** And if you are already happy enough, keep doing whatever it is you've been doing. And please, write a book to share your secret sauce with others. Then let me know when it's complete so I can read it, too.

# Bibliography

## Eat Up

Oliver, Jamie. *Cook with Jamie*. New York: The Penguin Group, 2007.

Neal, Moreton. *Remembering Bill Neal*. The University of North Carolina Press, 2004.

Oliver, Jamie. *The Naked Chef Takes Off*. The Penguin Group, 2000.

"Olive Oil's Health Benefits," http://www.healingdaily.com/detoxification-diet/olive-oil.htm (accessed July 1, 2009)

*Eat Smart with Ellie Krieger*. The Taunton Press, 2009.

Carlson O, Martin B, Stote KS, Golden E, Maudsley S, Najjar SS, Ferrucci L, Ingram DK, Longo DL, Rumpler WV, Baer DJ, Egan J, Mattson MP. "Impact of reduced meal frequency without caloric restriction on glucose regulation in healthy, normal-weight middle-aged men and women." *Metabolism* (December 2007), http://www.ncbi.nlm.nih.gov/sites/entrez?Db=pubmed&Cmd=ShowDetailView&TermToSearch=17998028&ordinalpos=1&itool=EntrezSystem2.PEntrez.Pubmed.Pubmed_ResultsPanel.Pubmed_RVDocSum.

Fitness and Nutrition Resource blog. "Skipping Meals and Metabolism." http://fitnessonline.blogspot.com/2007/12/skipping-meals-and-metabolism.html (December 26, 2007)

"Diet Tip: Skipping Meals." http://www.fitsugar.com/763935 (accessed November 2007).

Hedlund, Laurie, L.P.N. "Speed up Your Metabolism." http://www.consumeraffairs.com/nutrition/metab_speed.html (accessed July 1, 2009).

Garten, Ina. *The Barefoot Contessa Cookbook*. New York: Clarkson Potter, 1999.

The Moosewood Collective. *New Recipes from Moosewood Restaurant*. Berkeley, California: Ten Speed Press, 1987.

Vidalia Onion Committee. http://www.vidaliaonion.org/ (accessed July 1, 2009).

Wilson, Haley. "Simply Satisfying." *Cuisine at Home*. December 2008.

"Brown Rice vs White Rice." http://www.greenlivingtips.com/articles/94/1/Brown-rice-vs-white-rice.html, April 2007

"Advantages and Disadvantages of Being Vegetarian." http://www.allhealthsite.com/advantages-and-disadvantages-of-being-vegetarian.html, November 2008.

"Health Concerns about Meat." http://www.askdrsears.com/html/4/T043500.asp (accessed July 1, 2009).

Driver, Dustin. "Healthiest Meats." http://www.askmen.com/sports/foodcourt_150/184_eating_well.html (accessed July 1, 2009).

"Nutrition: How to Make Healthier Food Choices." http://familydoctor.org/online/famdocen/home/healthy/food/general-nutrition/297.html (accessed July 1, 2009).

Mayo Clinic staff. "Omega-3 in fish: How eating fish helps your heart." http://www.mayoclinic.com/health/omega-3/HB00087 (accessed July 1, 2009).

"Old Fashioned Caramel Layer Cake." *Cooking Light*. December 1999.

## Shape Up

"The Five Components of Physical Fitness." http://www.health-and-fitness-source.com/5-components-of-physical-fitness.html (accessed July 1, 2009).

"The 5 Components of Physical Fitness." http://www.lifetime-fitness-routines.com/componentsofphysicalfitness.html (accessed July 1, 2009).

Siller, Greg. "How to Improve Your 1-on-1 Battles with Muscular Strength and Endurance Training." http://www.prolearning.com/hockey/strength.htm (accessed July 1, 2009).

"Find out How to Develop your Muscular Endurance."http://www.fitnesshealthzone.com/exercises/find-out-how-to-develop-your-muscular-endurance/ (accessed July 1, 2009).

"Benefits of Yoga." http://www.healthandyoga.com/html/yoga/Benefits.html (accessed July 1, 2009).

"The Benefits of Stretching." http://www.functional-fitness-facts.com/benefits-of-stretching.html (accessed July 1, 2009).

Mayo Clinic staff. "Stretching: Focus on Flexibility." http://www.mayoclinic.com/health/stretching/HQ01447_ (accessed July 1, 2009).

Cook, Michelle. "The 12 Step Program to Healing Injuries." http://energyeffect.com/Articles/Article_12_Step_Program_to_Heal_Sports_Injuries.htm (accessed July 1, 2009).

Bedeaux, Jeff. "3 Biggest Benefits of Strength Training."_http://health.learninginfo.org/benefits-strength-training.htm (accessed July 1, 2009).

Mayo Clinic staff. "Strength training: Get stronger, leaner and healthier." http://www.mayoclinic.com/health/strength-training/ HQ01710 (accessed July 1, 2009).

"Should I Use Free Weights or Weight Machines? Weight Training Basics from Answer Fitness." http://www.answerfitness.com/91/ free-weights-weight-machines-weight-training-basics-answer-fitness/, April 5, 2008.

## Live It Up

Grogan, John. *Marley and Me.* New York: HarperCollins Publishers, 2005.

Shriver, Maria. *Just Who Will You Be?* New York: Hyperion, 2008.

*Jerry Maguire.* Directed by Cameron Crowe. 139 min. Gracie Films, TriStar Pictures, 1996.

*Spanglish.* Directed by James L. Brooks. 131 min. Gracie Films, Columbia Pictures, 2004.

# BUY A SHARE OF THE FUTURE IN YOUR COMMUNITY

These certificates make great holiday, graduation and birthday gifts that can be personalized with the recipient's name. The cost of one S.H.A.R.E. or one square foot is $54.17. The personalized certificate is suitable for framing and will state the number of shares purchased and the amount of each share, as well as the recipient's name. The home that you participate in "building" will last for many years and will continue to grow in value.

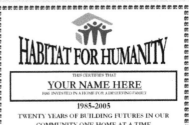

**Here is a sample SHARE certificate:**

## YES, I WOULD LIKE TO HELP!

*I support the work that Habitat for Humanity does and I want to be part of the excitement! As a donor, I will receive periodic updates on your construction activities but, more importantly, I know my gift will help a family in our community realize the dream of homeownership. **I would like to SHARE in your efforts against substandard housing in my community!** (Please print below)*

PLEASE SEND ME _____ SHARES at $54.17 EACH = $ $_____

*In Honor Of:* _____

*Occasion: (Circle One)*   HOLIDAY     BIRTHDAY     ANNIVERSARY

    OTHER: _____

*Address of Recipient:* _____

*Gift From:* _____ *Donor Address:* _____

*Donor Email:* _____

**I AM ENCLOSING A CHECK FOR $ $_____ PAYABLE TO HABITAT FOR HUMANITY OR PLEASE CHARGE MY VISA OR MASTERCARD** *(CIRCLE ONE)*

Card Number _____ Expiration Date: _____

Name as it appears on Credit Card _____ Charge Amount $ _____

Signature _____

Billing Address _____

Telephone # Day _____ Eve _____

**PLEASE NOTE:** Your contribution is tax-deductible to the fullest extent allowed by law.
**Habitat for Humanity • P.O. Box 1443 • Newport News, VA 23601 • 757-596-5553**
**www.HelpHabitatforHumanity.org**